English for Anatomy and Mind

髙木久代──編著

講談社

執筆者一覧

編著者

髙木 久代
鈴鹿医療科学大学保健衛生学部 教授（6，8，12章）

著者

山下 道世
鈴鹿医療科学大学看護学部 助教（1，3，11章）

平井 聡子
鈴鹿医療科学大学保健衛生学部 助教（2，9，10章）

服部 しのぶ
鈴鹿医療科学大学薬学部 教授（4，5，7章）

西田 圭吾
鈴鹿医療科学大学薬学部 教授（7章）

中西 健二
鈴鹿医療科学大学保健衛生学部 准教授（9章）

英文監修

Katherine Jordan Michels
鈴鹿医療科学大学保健衛生学部 助教

はじめに

　今日，日本においては高齢化が進み，高齢化の割合は世界一であるといわれています。加齢とともに様々な病気や怪我にみまわれることから逃れることはできません。医療分野においても，高齢化にともなう疾患の複雑化により高度な医療の必要性とともに，患者の体の一部分だけを治療するのではなく体全体を治療するホリスティックな治療が重要になっています。さらにインターネット社会では情報があふれ，体とともに心の状態が脅かされることが多くなっています。「心と身体は結びついている」という考えである「心身一如」があります。心の健全さは身体によい影響を及ぼす，その逆も然りです。私たちはこの考えに基づき体の健康とともに心の健康も考える必要があります。

　医療系の学生達の専攻は，英語ではなく各医療分野になります。英語を専攻しない学生が英語を積極的に学習するには強い動機づけが必要になります。そのため，将来医療系専門職で使える特殊な目的のための英語を学習する必要があります。本書は，解剖等にはじまり医療の専門的な語彙や内容についても英語で伝えられるよう実践的に学習できるように作成しています。さらに英語理解には不可欠な基本的な文法説明，読解練習問題等も加えています。

　本書は解剖，生理学を英語で学ぶ従来の英語教科書ではなく，「心身一如」の考えに基づき，心の問題や薬，ボランティア，薬膳等多岐にわたる話題を提供しています。さらに各章の最後にactivityを設けました。active-leaningの考えにより，各章を学び理解したのち，各自が提示された問題について考えて調べ，発表をします。この「特定の問題について自分で考え，発表する」活動の訓練は，チーム医療の中で仕事をするとき，カンファレンス等で役に立つことでしょう。

　今後，世界はさらにグローバル化が進み英語が今まで以上に必要になるでしょう。医療人として日本国内の外国人の対応のため，また海外で勤務するには医療の知識とともにコミュニケーションの手段として英語が必要になります。本書で英語語彙，文法の基礎，医療以外の知識を幅広く学んでいただき，将来の役に立てていただくことを願っています。

　最後に，本書を出版することができましたのは㈱講談社サイエンティフィクの三浦洋一郎様をはじめ，皆様のご支援のおかげでございます。心より感謝申し上げます。

2025年4月　著者一同

Contents

はじめに ——————————————————————— iii

Chapter **1** Blood ——————————————————— 1

Chapter **2** The Cardiovascular System ————————— 9

Chapter **3** The Respiratory System ————————— 17

Chapter **4** The Digestive System ——————————— 26

Chapter **5** The Urinary System ——————————— 34

Chapter **6** The Skeletal System (Bones, joints, and ligaments) ——— 42

Chapter **7** Food-Drug Interactions ————————— 52

Chapter **8** Yakuzen ——————————————— 59

Chapter **9** Stress ———————————————— 68

Chapter **10** Mindfulness ————————————— 76

Chapter **11** Broaden Your Horizons ————————— 84

Chapter **12** Volunteer Activity ——————————— 93

参考文献 ——————————————————————— 100

索引 ———————————————————————— 104

Chapter 1

Blood

血液成分とそれぞれの成分の役割について学びます。

Introduction

以下は血液を成分別に示した図です。1〜8に入る語句を選択肢から選んで空欄に記入しましょう。

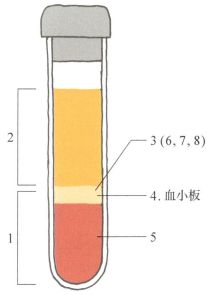

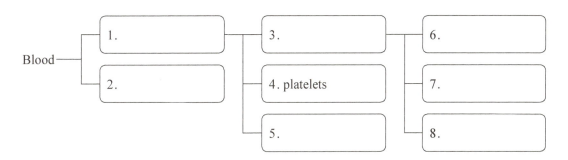

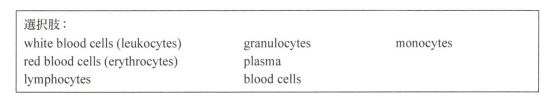

選択肢：

white blood cells (leukocytes)	granulocytes	monocytes
red blood cells (erythrocytes)	plasma	
lymphocytes	blood cells	

1-1. Dialogue

Mari（M）が，がんについての講義を受けた後，Haruto（H）と昼食をとっているところです。

M: Did you know that about 5,000 cancer cells are produced in the body every day, even in healthy people?

H: That many!? So why is it that only one in two Japanese people develop cancer, and not everyone?

M: It's because natural killer (NK) cells attack cancer cells. They are a type of leukocyte called lymphocytes. However, if a person's immune system becomes weakened, some cancer cells may survive and develop into cancer.

H: I see! Speaking of that, I've heard that laughing can help boost our immune system.

M: That's right! Research shows that laughing activates NK cells. Laughing can even help lower blood pressure. In addition, in patients with diabetes, it may help to lower after-meal blood sugar spikes and HbA1c levels.

H: Laughing must be very good for our health! However, life is not all fun and games. I once read that 4-year-olds laugh 300 times a day, while 40-year-olds only laugh 300 times in two and a half months.

M: We may laugh less as we grow older, but don't worry! Even a fake smile can provide health benefits.

H: Really? I'll try smiling then.

---

cancer cell　がん細胞

it is because〜
〜だからだ

natural killer cell
ナチュラルキラー細胞

leukocyte　白血球

lymphocyte　リンパ球

immune system　免疫系

develop into〜
〜に発展する

speaking of〜
〜と言えば

blood pressure　血圧

diabetes　糖尿病

blood sugar spike
血糖値の急上昇

HbA1c level
ヘモグロビンA1c値

must　〜に違いない

Point 💡 助動詞 must

助動詞のmustには「〜しなければならない」と「〜に違いない」という2つの用法があります。

例1：You must take your medicine as prescribed.
　　　あなたは処方されたとおりに薬を飲まなければならない。

例2：Laughing must be very good for our health!
　　　笑うことは私たちの健康にとても良いに違いない。

※否定文にする場合はdon't have to（〜する必要がない）を用いるので注意してください。
※must notの意味は，「〜してはならない（禁止）」と「〜のはずがない」の2つです。

Drill ✎

空欄に入る適切な語句を選択肢から選び記号で書きなさい。

1. A: I'm going to donate blood this weekend.
　　B: (　　　) donating blood, did you know there's a shortage at the blood bank?

2. The condition may (　　　) chronic pain, if left untreated.

3. The patient's test results show high blood sugar levels. It (　　　) be diabetes.

4. A: I bruise easily these days.
　　B: (　　　) your platelet count might be low.

5. (　　　) help protect your body from infections.

(a) must	(b) leukocytes	(c) speaking of
(d) that might be because	(e) develop into	(f) cancer cells

Chapter 1 Blood **3**

Questions and Answers

会話文を読み，次の問に英語で答えなさい。

1. Roughly how many cancer cells are produced every day?
   _____

2. What are natural killer (NK) cells and what do they do?
   _____

3. What are three benefits of laughing?
   _____

1-2. Reading

Vocabulary

arterial blood	動脈血	lymphocyte	リンパ球
basophil	好塩基球	monocyte	単球
blood cell	血球	mortality rate	死亡率
blood volume	血液量	neutrophil	好中球
bone marrow	骨髄	nutrient	栄養素
carbon dioxide	二酸化炭素	oxygenate	〜を酸素化する
circulate	循環する	pathogen	病原体
coagulation factor	凝固因子	phagocytize	貪食する
component	成分	plasma	血漿
concentration	濃度	platelet	血小板
draw	抜き出す	pulse oximeter	血中酸素濃度計
electrolyte	電解質	red blood cell (RBC)	赤血球
eosinophil	好酸球	tissue	組織
granulocyte	顆粒球	transfuse	輸血する
hematopoietic stem cell	造血幹細胞	transfusion	輸血
hemoglobin	ヘモグロビン	venous blood	静脈血
hemostasis	止血	waste product	老廃物
injury	外傷	white blood cell (WBC)	白血球

4

Do you know how many liters of blood circulate throughout your body? The blood volume of an adult is approximately 8% of their body weight. For example, in a person weighing 55 kg, roughly 4.5 liters of blood flow through them. This is equivalent to four and a half 1-liter milk cartons.

Blood consists of blood cells and plasma. The former accounts for about 45% of the total blood volume and includes red blood cells (RBCs), white blood cells (WBCs), and platelets. Blood cells originate from hematopoietic stem cells in the bone marrow. The latter accounts for about 55% of the total blood volume and consists of water, organic substances, and electrolytes. Let's take a closer look at these components and what roles they play.

The number of red blood cells is approximately 4 million per cubic millimeter of blood. Hemoglobin, the main component of red blood cells, contains iron, which gives blood its signature scent. The iron in hemoglobin binds with oxygen in the lungs, transporting it from the heart to body tissues. Oxygenated arterial blood is bright red, whereas venous blood is dark red due to its higher carbon dioxide content. Pulse oximeters utilize this color difference to measure the oxygen concentration in arterial blood. These devices can be attached to a finger to determine whether enough oxygen is being supplied without drawing any blood, making them very convenient.

The number of white blood cells is about 1/500 that of red blood cells. White blood cells consist of three types: granulocytes, which include neutrophils, eosinophils, and basophils; lymphocytes, which include T cells, B cells, and NK cells; and monocytes. White blood cells are immune cells that protect the body from pathogens such as viruses and bacteria. Neutrophils, the most numerous type of white blood cells, for instance, phagocytize and eliminate pathogens.

The number of platelets is about 1/25 that of red blood cells. The main function of platelets is hemostasis. Hemostasis involves multiple processes and various coagulation factors, with platelets being involved in primary hemostasis. It is known that people with blood type O have about 25% lower blood concentrations of a certain factor involved in hemostasis compared to those with other blood types. In fact, a study by Takayama et al. (2018) suggest that their mortality rate is more than twice as high as that of individuals with other blood types when they suffer severe injuries.

be equivalent to〜
〜と同等である

consist of〜
〜で構成されている

account for〜
〜を占める

originate from〜
〜に由来する

bind with〜
〜と結合する

transport O from A to B
OをAからBに運ぶ

due to〜　〜のために

whether SV
SVかどうか

protect O from〜
Oを〜から守る

such as〜　〜のような

be involved in〜
〜に関与する

compared to〜
〜に比べて

A is X times as 原級 as B
AはBのX倍原級だ

Plasma is a yellowish, transparent liquid composed mostly of water, with the remainder consisting of proteins, sugars, lipids, electrolytes, and waste products. Plasma transports nutrients to various parts of the body and collects waste products.

be composed of〜
〜で構成されている

In summary, blood is composed of various components, each with different roles. This is why, in transfusions, component transfusions are performed instead of whole blood transfusions, ensuring that only the necessary components are transfused.

instead of〜
〜の代わりに

Point 比較構文「as 原級 as」

「as 原級 as」は，「同じくらい〜」という意味です。
　　例1：This mountain is as high as that one.
　　　　この山はあの山と同じくらい高い。

「X times as 原級 as」は，「X倍の〜」という意味です。
　　例2：This mountain is twice as high as that one.
　　　　この山はあの山の2倍の高さである。

Drill

次の英文の［　　］内の語句を並び替えて，日本語訳に合う英文にしなさい。

1. White blood cells ［ from / the body / infections / protect ］.
　　白血球は，感染から身体を守る。
　　_____

2. Hemoglobin ［ the lungs / involved / in / is / oxygen / binding / in ］.
　　ヘモグロビンは，肺での酸素結合に関与している。
　　_____

3. Pulmonary veins ［ to / from / oxygen-rich blood / transport / the heart / the lungs ］.
　　肺静脈は，酸素の豊富な血液を肺から心臓に運ぶ。
　　_____

4. The test results will confirm ［ have / you / anemia / whether ］.
　　検査結果から貧血かどうかが判明する。
　　_____

5. ［ of / for / the body / 60％ / accounts / water ］ in adults.
　　水分は，成人の身体の60％を占める。
　　_____

Summary 📝

1～6に入る適切な語句を選択肢から選び，本文の要約を完成させなさい。

血液は1) _____ と2) _____ から成る。1) _____ は赤血球，白血球，血小板で構成され，血液量の約45％を占める。2) _____ は電解質や有機物が含まれる黄色い液体で，血液の約55％を占める。血液の成分にはそれぞれ重要な役割がある。ヘモグロビンを含む赤血球は，全身に3) _____ を運搬している。白血球は顆粒球，リンパ球，単球で構成され，病原体に対する4) _____ の機能をもつ。血小板は5) _____ に関係している。血漿は身体の各部分に6) _____ を運び，老廃物を回収する。このように血液の成分およびそれらの役割は多岐に渡る。

| 選択肢： | 酸素 | 一次止血 | 血球 | 栄養 | 免疫防御 | 血漿 |

Questions and Answers 🅠🅐

本文を読み，次の問に英語で答えなさい。

1. How many liters of blood circulate throughout your body?

_____

2. Why is venous blood dark red?

_____

3. What is the role of neutrophils?

_____

4. What is the main component of plasma?

_____

5. Why are component transfusions performed?

_____

Activity

血液や血管の健康の維持には，どのようなことが重要でしょうか。血液または血管のどちら
かを選び，調べてまとめましょう。

What is important for maintaining healthy blood and blood vessels? (Choose either "healthy blood" or "healthy blood vessels.")
1.
2.
3.
4.
5.

Chapter 2
The Cardiovascular System

心臓伝導系や血液循環について学びます。

Introduction

以下は心臓の解剖図です。1〜6に入る語句を，選択肢から選んで空欄に記入しましょう。

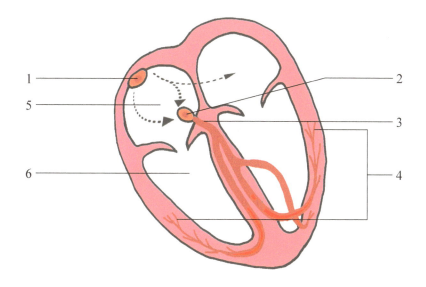

1.
2.
3.
4.
5.
6.

選択肢：
Purkinje fibers   right ventricle   left ventricle
right atrium   atrioventricular node   left atrium
sinoatrial node   bundle of His

2-1. Dialogue

Sara（S）と Riku（R）がアルバイト中に話しています。

S: Do you know how many times your heart beats in a day?

R: It varies from person to person, but I've heard it averages about 70 times per minute. If you calculate it based on 70 beats per minute, that comes out to over 100,000 beats per day.

based on～　～に基づいて

come out to　～になる

S: That means our hearts beat 36.5 million times a year. If a person lives to be 80, their heart will beat nearly 3 billion times!

R: That's an incredible number! It's astonishing to think that even when we're asleep, our heart never stops beating. What powers these heartbeats anyway? What keeps them constantly pumping?

S: I'd sure love to know! And while I hope they keep beating forever, I often hear about cardiac arrest on the news. If we ever encounter someone at school or work who has fallen unconscious and isn't breathing, what should we do?

cardiac arrest　心停止

fall unconscious
意識を失う

R: Last week, in a mandatory medical program for first-year students at my university, I learned how to perform CPR (Cardiopulmonary Resuscitation) and use an AED (Automated External Defibrillator). At first, it was nerve-wracking and tough, but I managed to learn how to do it correctly.

perform CPR
心肺蘇生法を行う

AED
自動体外式除細動器

S: That sounds like a great skill to have! If I ever get the chance, I'd love to learn it too. By the way, what specifically did you learn?

R: First, you must call out loudly for help, and then dial 119. Next, while waiting for the paramedics to arrive, check if there is an AED available. If there is, attach one pad to the upper right chest and the other to the lower left side of the chest to deliver a shock. If there is no AED available, place your hands one over the other on the center of the person's chest and press down about 5 cm at

call out loudly for help
大声で助けを呼ぶ

the paramedics　救急隊

attach it to　～に装着する

10

a steady rate of 100~120 compressions per minute.

S: That certainly sounds tough, but if there's even a small chance it could save someone's life, I want to train regularly.

at a steady rate
一定の速さで

Point 💡 過去分詞の副詞的用法

based on は「〜に基づいて」という意味の句で，ここでは過去分詞 based + 前置詞 on の形で，副詞的に使われています。

例1：When we choose a book based on the cover, we may make a mistake.
　　　表紙に基づいて本を選ぶと，間違えることがある。

例2：She made a decision based on the available data.
　　　彼女は利用可能なデータに基づいて決定した。

Drill ✏️

空欄に入る適切な語句を選択肢から選び，記号で書きなさい。

1. When encountering an emergency, the first step is to (　　　) and contact emergency services by dialing 119.

2. While waiting for (　　　) to arrive, it is crucial to check whether an (　　　) is available.

3. If an AED is available, one pad should be (　　　) to the upper right chest and the other to the lower left chest before proceeding to (　　　).

4. If no AED is available, place one hand over the other in the center of the chest and apply chest compressions at a depth of approximately 5 cm (　　　) of 100~120 compressions per minute.

(a) the paramedics	(b) call out loudly for help	(c) AED
(d) at a steady rate	(e) perform CPR	(f) attached

Chapter 2　The Cardiovascular System　**11**

Questions and Answers

会話文を読み，次の問に英語で答えなさい。

1. Roughly how many times does the heart beat in a month?
   _____

2. When you see a person who has fallen unconscious, what is the first action you should take?
   _____

3. Where on the body should you attach place an AED?
   _____

2-2. Reading

Vocabulary

aorta	大動脈	inferior vena cava (IVC)	下大静脈
arterial blood	動脈血	metabolic waste product	代謝廃棄物
atrioventricular node	房室結節	oxygen	酸素
atrium	心房	pacemaker	ペースメーカー
bundle branch	束枝または脚	peripheral tissue	末梢組織
bundle of His	ヒス束	pulmonary artery	肺動脈
carbon dioxide	二酸化炭素	pulmonary circulation	肺循環
cardiac conduction system	心臓伝導系	Purkinje fiber	プルキンエ線維
cardiovascular	心血管の	relaxation	弛緩
contraction	収縮	sinoatrial node	洞房結節
electrical activity	電気活動	superior vena cava (SVC)	上大静脈
electrical impulse	電気インパルス（電気的刺激）	systemic circulation	体循環
electrocardiogram (ECG)	心電図	vein	静脈
heartbeat	心拍	ventricle	心室

The heart is located on the left side of the chest and is about the size of a fist. The heart is composed of four chambers: the right atrium, right ventricle, left ventricle, and left atrium. These four chambers rhythmically cycle between contraction and relaxation to circulate blood. This rhythm is created by what is called the cardiac conduction system. The cardiac conduction system consists of five parts: the sinoatrial node, the atrioventricular node, the bundle of His, the left and right bundle branches, and the Purkinje fibers.

The sinoatrial node, also known as the pacemaker, is made up of specialized cardiac cells. What is so unique about this node is how it automatically generates electrical impulses without any command from the brain or other sources, and causes the heart to contract. This process begins when the sinoatrial node in the right atrium generates "electricity," which then transmits an impulse through the other parts in the order mentioned above. This prompts the Purkinje fibers to send electricity throughout the entire heart like a network.

Thanks to the heart's constant pumping action, blood circulates throughout the body. This process of circulation, where blood leaves the heart, passes through the body's capillaries, and returns to the heart, is called systemic circulation. On the other hand, the process where blood leaves the heart, passes through the lungs, and returns to the heart, is called pulmonary circulation.

In systemic circulation, oxygen-rich arterial blood flows through the arteries, while venous blood containing waste products like carbon dioxide flows through the veins. In pulmonary circulation, venous blood flows through the pulmonary artery, where carbon dioxide is exchanged for oxygen in the lungs. This newly oxygenated blood then returns to the heart through the pulmonary veins. Through circulation, not only oxygen but also nutrients are delivered throughout the body, while metabolic waste products are carried away from the peripheral tissues for removal.

The aorta is the largest artery, and the inferior vena cava (IVC) is the largest vein. The pathway of the aorta begins at the heart and travels down through the chest and abdomen, sending blood throughout the body. The IVC collects blood from the lower part of the body and sends it straight to the heart.

There is also another large and important vein called the superior vena cava (SVC). The SVC is responsible for collecting and returning deoxygenated blood from the upper part of the body to the heart.

To examine cardiovascular function, an electrocardiogram (ECG) is used to measure the electrical activity of the heart. It provides a graphic representation of how the heart beats and helps assess how well the heart is functioning. Heartbeats are recorded by an ECG machine and displayed as a series of waves on a graph. An ECG is quick, painless, and provides important information about heart health.

be responsible for
〜の責任がある

assess how well the heart is functioning
心臓がどれほど機能しているかを評価する

be recorded by
〜によって記録される

be displayed as
a series of waves
一連の波として表示される

Point 💡 受動態と能動態

be composed of は「〜から構成される」という意味で，受動態の形で使われます。consist of は「〜から成る」という意味で，能動態の形で使われます。2つの用法を注意して使い分けましょう。

例1：Water is composed of hydrogen and oxygen.
　　　水は水素と酸素から構成されている。

例2：A week consists of seven days.
　　　1週間は7日から成る。

Summary 📄

1〜5に入る適切な語句を選択肢から選び，本文の要約を完成させなさい。

　「心臓伝導系」は，洞房結節，房室結節，1)＿＿＿＿＿＿，左右の脚，プルキンエ線維の5つの部分から成り立っている。2)＿＿＿＿＿＿は「ペースメーカー」と呼ばれ，脳からの3)＿＿＿＿＿＿電気的インパルスを生成し，それが心臓全体に伝わる。
　体循環では，4)＿＿＿＿＿＿を豊富に含んだ動脈血が動脈を通り，一方で二酸化炭素などの廃棄物を含んだ静脈血が静脈を通る。肺循環では，5)＿＿＿＿＿＿が肺動脈を通り，肺で二酸化炭素が酸素と交換される。

選択肢：	酸素	ヒス束	静脈血	動脈血
	洞房結節	指令により	指令なしに	房室結節

Drill

次の英文の［　］内の語句を並び替えて，日本語訳に合う英文にしなさい。

1. The ［ four / human / heart / composed / is / chambers / of ］.
   人間の心臓は，4つの「部屋」で構成されている。

   _____

2. The sinoatrial node ［ as / pacemaker of / the heart / known / the natural / is ］.
   洞房結節は，心臓の自然なペースメーカーとして知られている。

   _____

3. The nervous system ［ responsible / increasing / for / the heart rate / is ］.
   神経系は心拍数の増加を担っている。

   _____

4. The nervous system ［ a signal / causing / in / , / heart rate / an increase / sends ］.
   神経系は信号を送信し，それが心拍数の増加を引き起こす。

   _____

5. The patient's ［ heart rhythm / recorded / by / abnormal / was ］ an electrocardiogram (ECG).
   患者の異常な心拍リズムは，心電図（ECG）によって記録された。

   _____

Questions and Answers

本文を読み，次の問に英語で答えなさい。

1. Why is the sinoatrial node considered unique in its function?
   _____

2. How does the sinoatrial node generate electrical impulses for the heart?
   _____

3. Where does systemic circulation send blood after it leaves the heart?
   _____

4. What does an electrocardiogram (ECG) measure?
   _____

Activity

Heart Disease Prevention Campaign（心臓病予防キャンペーン）として，心臓病を予防する方法を以下の順序に従い1枚のポスターにまとめてみましょう。

1. 予防したい心臓疾患を選びましょう。
2. その疾患に対する予防法を調べましょう。
3. 調べた予防法を，自分や家族が実際に取り組みやすい方法にアレンジしましょう。
4. キャンペーンの目的が一目でわかるような，インパクトのあるポスターを英語で作りましょう。

Chapter 3
The Respiratory System

呼吸器系の区分とそれぞれの役割について学びます。

Introduction

以下は呼吸器系を表す図です。1〜10に入る語句を選択肢から選んで空欄に記入しましょう。

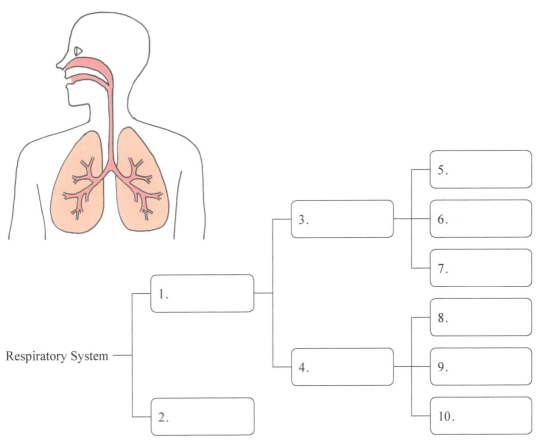

※alveoliは10の末端にあります。

選択肢：
airways
bronchi
bronchioles
larynx
lower respiratory tract
lungs
nasal cavity
pharynx
upper respiratory tract
trachea

3-1. Dialogue

Riku（R）と Yoko（Y）は登山を終えて山頂にたどり着いたところです。

R: What a beautiful day today! The weather forecast said that neither pollen nor fine particulate matter (PM2.5) would be a problem today.

neither A nor B～
A も B も～ない

Y: It feels great! Did you know that the United Nations (UN) designated September 7 as the International Day of Clean Air for Blue Skies?

designate　定める

R: I didn't! Why is that?

Y: According to the World Health Organization (WHO), ambient and domestic air pollution are serious global issues. They don't only affect global warming but also pose a threat to people's health. So, the UN is working to raise awareness and improve the current situation.

ambient　環境の

domestic　家庭の

air pollution　大気汚染

pose a threat to～
～を脅かす

raise awareness　意識を高める

R: Wow, how serious is it?

on top of that　そのうえ

be responsible for～
～の原因になっている

Y: The WHO says that 99% of the world's population lives in areas with air pollution levels that exceed the WHO guidelines set in 2021. On top of that, air pollution is responsible for 6.7 million premature deaths every year.

premature death　早死に

in detail　詳細に

pollutant　汚染物質

carbon monoxide
一酸化炭素

R: Can you explain that in more detail?

respiratory　呼吸器の

chronic obstructive
pulmonary disease
慢性閉塞性肺疾患

Y: Sure. Pollutants such as PM2.5, carbon monoxide, and ozone cause respiratory illnesses such as chronic obstructive pulmonary disease (COPD), lung cancer, and acute respiratory infections. Moreover, PM2.5 can enter the bloodstream and contribute to ischemic heart disease and stroke.

lung cancer　肺がん

acute respiratory infection
急性呼吸器感染症

bloodstream　血流

contribute to～　～の一因となる

ischemic heart disease
虚血性心疾患

R: That means that the impact of air pollution goes beyond the lungs and affects the heart and brain as well.

stroke　卒中

Y: Each of us should take an interest and start taking action whenever we can.

take an interest
興味を持つ

R: You are absolutely right! I'll pledge to stop driving to school and start using both public transportation and a bicycle instead.

absolutely　まったく

pledge to〜　〜を誓う

public transportation
公共交通機関

Y: That's a great idea! In countries like the Netherlands and Denmark, well-developed cycling infrastructure has led to high rates of bicycle usage.

infrastructure
社会基盤施設

R: That makes sense!

neither A nor B

neither A nor B は「AもBもどちらも〜ない」という意味です。not は含まれませんが，否定の意味になります。なお，動詞の形は，主語Bに合わせます。

例1：Neither injections nor <u>medications</u> were available.
　　　注射も薬も入手できなかった。

　　　同じ種類の接続詞として，both A and B（AとBの両方）があります。この場合，動詞の形は主語 A and B に合わせます。

例2：Both <u>the doctor and the nurse</u> are attending the consultation with the patient.
　　　医師と看護師の両者が，患者との診察に立ち会っている。

Drill

空欄に入る適切な語句を選択肢から選び記号で書きなさい。

1. Air pollution (　　　) various respiratory diseases.

2. Respiratory infections may (　　　) the development of pneumonia.

3. The government launched a campaign to (　　　) about the harmful effects of smoking on lung health.

4. Long-term exposure to air pollutants (　　　) respiratory health.

5. The trachea is (　　　) a muscle nor a bone; it is made of cartilage.

| (a) raise awareness | (b) contribute to | (c) poses a threat to |
| (d) take an interest | (e) is responsible for | (f) neither |

Questions and Answers

会話文を読み，次の問に英語で答えなさい。

1. How serious of a problem is global air pollution?

2. What are five diseases caused by the air pollutants?

3. How can air pollution be reduced?

3-2. Reading

Vocabulary

airway	気道	humidify	湿度を与える
alveolus（複 alveoli）	肺胞	larynx	喉頭
breathe	息をする	lobe	葉（肺の）
bronchial tree	気管支樹	lower respiratory tract	下気道
bronchiole	細気管支	nasal cavity	鼻腔
bronchus（複 bronchi）	気管支	pharynx	咽頭
chest	胸部	sleep apnea	睡眠時無呼吸
chronic	慢性の	sleep disorder	睡眠障害
deficiency	欠乏	swallow	飲み込む
diaphragmatic	横隔膜の	symptom	症状
epiglottis	喉頭蓋	thoracic vertebra	胸椎
esophagus	食道	trachea	気管
expulsion	排出	tracheal cartilage	気管軟骨
foreign particle	異物	upper respiratory tract	上気道

The respiratory system is composed of the airways, alveoli, and lungs. The airways serve as the passage for air and are divided into the upper respiratory tract, which includes the nasal cavity, pharynx, and larynx, and the lower respiratory tract, which includes the trachea, bronchi, and bronchioles. The alveoli are located at the ends of the bronchioles in the lungs.

Let's first take a look at the upper respiratory tract. The nasal cavity warms and humidifies the incoming air, and its nasal hairs act as a filter for foreign particles. The next section is the pharynx, which connects to both the esophagus and the larynx. The esophagus carries food to the stomach, while the larynx is part of the respiratory system. The larynx contains the epiglottis, which functions as a

be composed of ～
～で構成されている

serve as～
～として機能する

be divided into～
～に分けられる

Chapter 3 The Respiratory System **21**

lid to prevent food from entering the trachea during swallowing.

Do you breathe in air through your nasal cavity when you breathe? A survey of 3,399 Japanese children aged 3 to 12 revealed that approximately 30% had lip seal insufficiency, suggesting a correlation with mouth breathing. You might be mouth breathing without even realizing, so be careful because mouth breathing can lead to symptoms such as dry mouth and bad breath. Additionally, people who breathe through their mouths tend to suffer from sleep disorders like sleep apnea. Some doctors also believe that mouth breathing is related to various diseases. One method to correct mouth breathing is mouth taping, a simple technique where mouth tape is applied during sleep.

Next, let's examine the lower respiratory tract, alveoli, and lungs. The trachea is a tube located in front of the esophagus, composed of 15 to 20 U-shaped tracheal cartilages. It is 10-15 cm long and 2.0-2.5 cm in diameter. The trachea splits into the left and right bronchi at the level of the fifth thoracic vertebra, behind the heart. The right and left bronchi differ in length and angle because the heart is positioned slightly to the left of the body's center. The right bronchus is 2.5 cm long and angles at 25 degrees from the trachea, while the left bronchus is 5 cm long and angles at 35 degrees. The bronchi enter the left and right lungs and branch 23 times before reaching the alveoli. They are collectively called the bronchial tree and help deliver air to over 300 million alveoli. The alveoli are responsible for the intake of oxygen and the expulsion of carbon dioxide. The lungs are asymmetrical, with the right lung having three lobes and the left lung having two lobes. The left lung is smaller than the right lung due to the heart's position.

Breathing occurs 12 to 20 times per minute. It is said that modern people experience shallow breathing due to stress, which can lead to chronic oxygen deficiency. If breathing is shallow, it becomes chest breathing, so it is important to practice diaphragmatic breathing to assure the intake of sufficient oxygen.

---

prevent O from 〜ing
Oが〜するのを防ぐ

lead to〜　〜につながる

suffer from〜　〜を患う

be related to〜
〜に関係している

split into〜
〜に分かれる

be responsible for〜
〜を担う

due to〜　〜が原因で

Point to不定詞

to 不定詞には，名詞的用法，形容詞的用法，副詞的用法の3つの用法があります。

1．名詞的用法：名詞の働きをする。

It is important to practice diaphragmatic breathing.
横隔膜呼吸を実践することは重要だ。
➡ 形式主語itに対する本当の主語（真主語）。

2．形容詞的用法：直前の名詞を修飾し，形容詞の働きをする。

One method to correct mouth breathing is mouth taping.
口呼吸を矯正する方法の1つは，マウステーピングだ。
➡ one method（名詞）を修飾している。

3．副詞的用法：動詞・形容詞・副詞や文を修飾し，副詞の働きをする。

It is important to practice diaphragmatic breathing to assure the intake of sufficient oxygen.
十分な酸素の取り込みを確実にするために，横隔膜呼吸を実践することが重要である。
➡ practice（動詞）を修飾している。

Drill

次の英文の［ ］内の語句を並び替えて，日本語訳に合う英文にしなさい。

1. The alveoli ［ facilitate / serve / gas exchange / that / as / tiny air sacs ］ in the lungs.
   肺胞は，肺のガス交換を促進する小さな気嚢として機能する。

2. Vaccination ［ seriously / from / can / us / help / ill / prevent / getting ］.
   ワクチン接種は，私たちが重症になるのを防ぐのに役立つ。

3. ［ can / to / to / exposure / prolonged / lead / air pollutants ］ chronic obstructive pulmonary disease (COPD).
   大気汚染物質に長期間さらされると，慢性閉塞性肺疾患につながる可能性がある。

4. More and more people ［ due / air / asthma / pollution / from / to / suffer ］.
   ますます多くの人が，大気汚染のために喘息で苦しんでいる。

5. Chronic coughing ［ related / as / may / conditions / bronchitis / be / such / to ］.
   慢性的な咳は，気管支炎などの疾患と関連しているかもしれない。

Summary 📄

1～6に入る適切な語句を選択肢から選び，本文の要約を完成させなさい。

　呼吸器系は気道と1) _____ および肺で構成されている。気道は上気道と下気道から成り，前者には，鼻腔，2) _____ ，喉頭が，後者には気管，3) _____ ，細気管支がそれぞれ含まれる。1)は3億個以上あり，そこでは4) _____ が行われる。口呼吸は様々な症状を引き起こすため，5) _____ を意識し，また，酸素不足にならないために胸式呼吸ではなく6) _____ を心がける。

選択肢：	腹式呼吸	肺胞	気管支	鼻呼吸	ガス交換	咽頭

Questions and Answers 🅠🅐

本文を読み，次の問に英語で答えなさい。

1. What are the roles of the nasal cavity?

　_____

2. What are some of the symptoms associated with mouth breathing?

　_____

3. Why do the right and left bronchi differ in length and angle?

　_____

4. What are the components of the bronchial tree?

　_____

5. What is the function of the alveoli?

　_____

Activity

国や地域または都道府県などを限定し，最近の大気汚染状況について調べ，まとめましょう。また20年前の状況と比較しましょう。

調査した場所：_____

最近の大気汚染状況

20年前の大気汚染状況

Chapter 4

The Digestive System

消化器系の解剖生理について学びます。

Introduction

以下は消化器系を示した図です。1〜8に入る語句を選択肢から選んで空欄に記入しましょう。

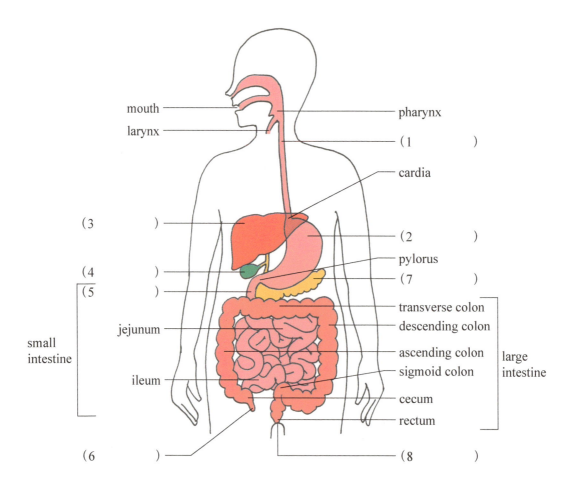

選択肢：

| esophagus | stomach | appendix | pancreas |
| gallbladder | duodenum | liver | anus |

4-1. Dialogue

Mr. Kato (K) と Ms. Mori (M) が話をしています。Ms. Mori は，最近職場を異動になり，健康状態の変化に気づきました。

K: Have you gotten used to the new workplace?

M: Yes, thank you. While I've been managing, my stomach hasn't been feeling well recently.

K: What's wrong?

M: It's strange. At first, I was constipated, so I took a laxative. After a while, I started having diarrhea and my bowels became loose.

K: I'm sorry to hear that. Are you alternating between constipation and diarrhea? I've heard that the stomach and intestines are easily affected by stress.

M: That might be it. Since I was suddenly transferred to a new department at work, my environment and relationships have changed, and I feel more tense with every passing day.

K: That could be the cause. I think environmental changes are more stressful than we realize.

M: Yes, you're right ... I think I'll go to the hospital soon.

get used to	～に慣れる
What's wrong?	どうしたのですか？
be constipated	便秘である
laxative	便秘薬
diarrhea	下痢
loose	ゆるい
alternate	行ったり来たりする
between A and B	AとBの間
be transferred to ～	～へ異動する
tense	緊張した
passing day	過ぎゆく1日1日
more ～ than ...	…よりもっと～

便秘と下痢を繰り返す症状は，もしかしたら過敏性腸症候群かもしれません。今回のように，環境の変化により，無意識に精神的なストレスが溜まり発症することがあります。まずは，医療機関やかかりつけ医の受診をしましょう。

Point 💡 現在完了形

I've been ... や I've heard that ... にみられる have + 過去分詞の形は，現在完了形といわれる表現です。過去のある時点から現在まで動作が継続していることや，経験，動作の完了などを表します。

例1：I've been managing a busy schedule. ➡ 現在完了進行形（継続）
多忙な予定を何とかこなしている。

例2：I've heard that he moved to a new workplace. ➡ 現在完了形（経験）
彼が新しい職場に異動したと聞いたことがある。

例3：The meeting has just finished. ➡ 現在完了形（完了）
ミーティングがちょうど終わった。

Drill ✏️

空欄に入る適切な語句を選択肢から選び記号で書きなさい。

1. I have (　　) that the construction of the building will finish next April.

2. My environment has (　　) since I got married and moved to this city.

3. We (　　) learned that we should respect individuals.

4. It is (　　) comfortable for me to be at home than to go out.

5. The score of the exam was much (　　) than I expected.

(a) have	(b) changed	(c) heard
(d) more	(e) higher	

Questions and Answers

会話文を読み，次の問に英語で答えなさい。

1. What symptoms does Ms. Mori have?
　_____

2. What could be the cause of these symptoms?
　_____

4-2.　Reading

Vocabulary

anus	肛門	ileum	回腸
appendix	虫垂	insulin	インスリン
bile	胆汁	intestine	腸
bloodstream	血流	islet of Langerhans	ランゲルハンス島
cardia	噴門	jejunum	空腸
cecum	盲腸	larynx	喉頭
colon	結腸	mucosa	粘膜
diaphragm	横隔膜	mucous membrane	粘膜
digestive fluid	消化液	pancreas	膵臓
digestive system	消化器系	pancreatic juice	膵液
duodenum	十二指腸	papilla	乳頭
endocrine gland	内分泌腺	portal vein	門脈
epiglottis	喉頭蓋	pylorus	幽門
esophagus	食道	rectum	直腸
exocrine fluid	外分泌液	saliva	唾液
feces	糞便	sigmoid colon	S状結腸
gallbladder	胆嚢	swallowing reflex	嚥下反射
gastric juice	胃液	villus	絨毛
glucagon	グルカゴン	windpipe	気管
hemorrhoid	痔		

Chapter 4　The Digestive System　29

Food is used for repairing cells and supplying them with energy. The digestive system helps the body digest food, absorb nutrients, and eliminate waste. Digestion involves converting food into a liquid form, allowing it to pass through the walls of the digestive tract and enter the bloodstream to be transported to cells.

The digestive process begins in the mouth. In the mouth, food is chewed and mixed with saliva, making it easier to swallow. The food then travels down the esophagus, a 25-30 cm long tube located behind the windpipe, to the stomach. Meanwhile, the epiglottis, part of the larynx, prevents food from entering the airway through the swallowing reflex. The esophagus leads to the cardia of the stomach, an organ that changes in volume depending on the amount of food it holds. The stomach secretes about 1,500 mL of gastric juice daily, where the food is broken down into a porridge-like consistency and then passed through the pylorus into the duodenum, a C-shaped structure that is the first part of the small intestine. In the duodenum, the highly acidic contents from the stomach are neutralized by alkaline secretions to protect the mucous membrane. Bile and pancreatic juice are added to initiate the primary digestion of nutrients. The duodenal mucosa has the major duodenal papilla, which regulates the flow of bile and pancreatic juice.

The small intestine, measuring about 6 meters long, is divided into the duodenum, jejunum, and ileum. The mucosa lining the walls of the small intestine is densely packed with villi, which increase the surface area to efficiently absorb nutrients. Approximately 2,400 mL of alkaline digestive fluid is secreted in the small intestine daily to promote digestion and nutrient absorption.

Nutrients are transported to the liver via the portal vein. The liver, located just below the diaphragm, has three primary functions: metabolism, the production and storage of bile (an exocrine fluid), and blood filtration. More than half of the bile produced by the liver is stored in the gallbladder for reuse in digestion. The pancreas, located near the gallbladder and behind the stomach, measures 14-18 cm in length. The exocrine glands of the pancreas secrete pancreatic juice, which aids in the digestion of sugars, proteins, and fats. The endocrine glands, known as the islets of Langerhans, secrete hormones such as insulin and glucagon.

The large intestine, the final part of the intestine, includes the

---

digest 消化する

absorb 吸収する

eliminate 排除する

convert... into〜
…を〜に変える

allow〜 to...
〜に…させる

chew かむ

located 位置している

depending on〜
〜によって

the amount of〜 〜の量

secrete 分泌する

porridge-like
おかゆのような

consistency 粘度

acidic 酸性の

alkaline アルカリ性の

regulate 制限する

be divided into〜
〜に分けられる

lining 内張り

be packed with〜
〜でいっぱいである

be transported to〜
〜へ運ばれる

via〜 〜経由で

filtration ろ過

in length 長さで

such as〜 〜のような

cecum with the appendix, ascending colon, transverse colon, descending colon, sigmoid colon, and rectum. The rectum is the last part of the large intestine, approximately 20 cm long, and opens to the outside of the body as the anus. The large intestine extracts water from the remaining food waste from the small intestine, forming feces. The mucosa of the anus is densely packed with veins, which are prone to bleeding due to hemorrhoids.

extract　抽出する

remaining　残っている

, forming〜
そして〜を形成する

be prone to〜
〜しがちである

due to〜　〜のせいで

The digestive system ranges from the mouth to the anus, through which waste exits the body.

Point 💡 関係副詞と関係代名詞の非制限用法

関係詞の前にカンマを置いて，先行詞の説明を加える用法で，前から順に訳していきます。

例1： The stomach secretes about 1,500 mL of gastric juice daily, where the food is broken down into a porridge-like consistency...
胃は毎日1,500 mL くらいの胃液を分泌し，そして，そこで（the stomach）食べ物がおかゆ状の粘度に分解される…

例2： The duodenal mucosa has the major duodenal papilla, which regulates the flow of bile and pancreatic juice.
十二指腸の粘膜には主に十二指腸乳頭があり，そして，それは（papilla）胆汁と膵液の流れを制限する。

Drill ✏

下記の文の空欄に，which か where か正しい方を書き入れなさい。

1. I moved to this city, (　　　　　) I got a new job.

2. She designed a dress, (　　　　　) looks like a Cinderella's.

3. He provided a part of his garden, (　　　　　) his friends can park their cars.

4. We gave children some cookies, (　　　　　) we baked for a charity.

5. There is a free space inside the building, (　　　　　) people enjoy chatting.

Chapter 4 The Digestive System **31**

Summary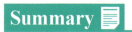

1〜7に入る適切な語句を選択肢から選び，本文の要約を完成させなさい。

　消化器官は，身体が食物を消化し，栄養を取り込み，老廃物を排出するのを助ける。まず，口に入った食物は咀嚼され唾液がかけられ，滑りやすくなって 1) ＿＿＿＿＿ へ送られる。1) ＿＿＿＿＿ は，2) ＿＿＿＿＿ の噴門へと続いており，そこで食物はおかゆ状に分解される。そして，次に，小腸（6メートルにも及ぶ）の最初の部分であるC字型の 3) ＿＿＿＿＿ へ送られる。そこで 4) ＿＿＿＿＿ と 5) ＿＿＿＿＿ が加えられ消化がさらに進み，粘膜に密集する絨毛に栄養が吸収される。その後，6) ＿＿＿＿＿ では，小腸から送られてきた食物の残りから水分が抜き取られ，7) ＿＿＿＿＿ が作られ，体外に排出される。

選択肢： 食道　　胃　　十二指腸　　胆汁　　膵液　　大腸　　糞便

Questions and Answers

本文を読み，次の問に英語で答えなさい。

1. What prevents aspiration?
   _____

2. What does the duodenal papilla do?
   _____

3. How much digestive juice is secreted in the small intestine daily?
   _____

4. Within which blood vessel do nutrients go through to the liver?
   _____

5. What is extracted in the large intestine?
   _____

Activity

1. 内分泌系と外分泌系の機能と構成について，膵臓やランゲルハンス島から分泌されるホルモンなどを例に挙げて，調べてみましょう。

2. 消化器系の代表的な疾患について，調べてみましょう。

1.

2.

Chapter 4 The Digestive System **33**

Chapter 5

The Urinary System

泌尿器系の解剖生理について学びます。

Introduction

以下は泌尿器系を示した図です。1〜8に入る語句を選択肢から選んで空欄に記入しましょう。

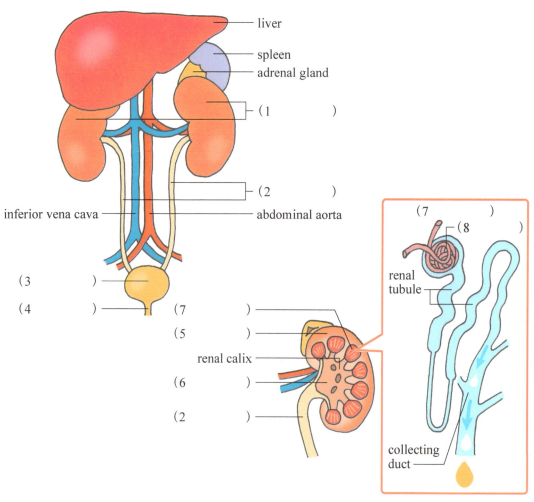

選択肢：			
kidney	urethra	ureter	bladder
cortex	renal pelvis	nephron	glomerulus

5-1. Dialogue

Mr. Kato（K）は急なひどい腹痛のため病院に運ばれ，MRI の検査をし，Dr. Yamada（Y）と話をしています。

Y: (Showing Mr. Kato the image) There's a shadow here that seems to be a stone. To pass it, you just need to drink plenty of fluids.

pass　通過する

K: I see. How much water should I drink?

Y: About two liters a day.

K: Oh. It's winter, so I don't usually drink much, but I'll try my best to drink more.

Y: There are also medications to help pass the stone more quickly. Would you like to take those?

K: For now, I'll try to pass it on my own by drinking a lot of water.

on my own　自分で

Y: The stone will likely pass within one to two months. If you bring in the stone that passed through, we can analyze what it's made of and determine its cause.

likely　おそらく

analyze　分析する

be made of〜
〜でできている

K: What does it look like when it comes out?

look like〜
〜のように見える

Y: It looks like a white *kompeito* (Japanese sugar candy) and varies in size.

vary in size
大きさに差がある

K: Oh, I see.

Y: If the stone hasn't passed by your next visit, we might consider using medication, but for today I'll just prescribe a painkiller.

consider 〜ing
〜することを検討する

prescribe　処方する

painkiller　鎮痛剤

K: Okay, thank you.

Chapter 5 The Urinary System　**35**

Note

　本会話に登場する患者さんは，ひどい腹痛がありMRIの画像に石が写っています。これは，尿路結石かもしれません。原因の1つとして，肉類の摂りすぎによりシュウ酸が増え，尿のカルシウムと結合して石が形成される，とも考えられます。野菜を多く摂り水分もしっかり補給し，運動もすることで予防できます。

Point　be made of と be made from

be made ofとbe made fromは，どちらも「～でできている」という意味ですが，若干使い方が異なります。ofは，原材料が目で見てわかるもの，一方，fromは，原材料が形を変えてわからなくなっている場合に使います。以下の例で確認しましょう。

例1：The desk is made of wood.
　　　その机は木でできている。

例2：Wine is made from grapes.
　　　ワインはブドウからできている。

Drill

下記の文の空欄に，ofかfromか正しい方を書き入れなさい。

1. This soup is made (　　　　) a pumpkin and potatoes.

2. Have you ever used a straw made (　　　　) paper?

3. It is heavy because it is made (　　　　) stones.

4. The butter is made (　　　　) milk.

5. Her ring is made (　　　　) gold.

Questions and Answers

会話文を読み，次の問に英語で答えなさい。

1. How will Mr. Kato pass the stone?
   _____

2. What will the stone look like?
   _____

5-2. Reading

Vocabulary

bladder	膀胱	renal corpuscle	腎小体
Bowman's capsule	ボーマン嚢	renal cortex	腎皮質
capillary	毛細血管	renal medulla	腎髄質
cluster	かたまり	renal pelvis	腎盂
collecting duct	集合管	renal tubule	尿細管
convoluted tubule	尿細管	renal vein	腎静脈
glomerulus（複 glomeruli）	糸球体	toxin	毒
kidney	腎臓	ureter	尿管
nephron	ネフロン（腎単位）	urethra	尿道
peristaltic movement	蠕動運動	urinary system	泌尿器系
peritoneum	腹膜	urinary tract	尿路
renal artery	腎動脈	urine	尿

The urinary system is a group of organs responsible for excreting waste products from the body. It is composed of two kidneys, two ureters, the bladder, and the urethra. The two kidneys, shaped like beans and each approximately 12 cm long, are located on the left and right sides of the body behind the peritoneum. Each

be responsible for ～
～の責任を負う，関与している

be composed of ～
～から成る

kidney has renal veins, renal arteries, and nerves entering it. The pathway through which urine passes is called the urinary tract, extending from the ureters to the bladder and urethra. Blood flows from the renal arteries through gradually narrowing small arteries, reaching structures called glomeruli, which consist of capillaries arranged in clusters. The blood exits each glomerulus through finer veins, ultimately leaving through a large renal vein.

The primary function of the kidneys is to regulate the volume and composition of urine in response to the body's condition and the intake and loss of water and salts, thereby maintaining a stable internal environment. Additional functions include blood filtration, the excretion of waste products produced in the body, the processing of drugs and harmful substances (toxins), blood pressure regulation, and the secretion of various hormones.

The kidney is divided into two regions: the outer cortex (renal cortex) and the inner medulla (renal medulla). The renal cortex contains renal corpuscles (glomeruli and Bowman's capsules) and renal tubules. The renal tubules in the cortex include structures like the proximal and distal convoluted tubules, which are important for filtration and reabsorption. The renal medulla contains straight tubules. The smallest functional unit of the kidney is called the nephron, where blood filtration and urine production occur. Each kidney contains about one million nephrons, consisting of a thin-walled structure (Bowman's capsule) that surrounds the glomerulus, the internal space of Bowman's capsule (Bowman's space), and a narrow tube (renal tubule) that drains fluid from Bowman's space. Urine from multiple renal tubules flows into the collecting ducts, eventually reaching the renal pelvis in the center of the kidney. Urine is formed in the kidney through a two-step process of glomerular filtration and tubular reabsorption. Approximately 200 liters of urine (primary urine) are filtered from the blood daily at the glomeruli, with 99% being reabsorbed into the bloodstream in the renal tubules. This results in about 1.5 liters of final urine. Urine is collected from multiple renal tubules into the collecting ducts.

The ureters are muscular tubes approximately 40 cm long, with the upper ends connected to the kidneys and the lower ends to the bladder. Urine produced in the kidneys is gradually transported through the ureters to the bladder by peristaltic movement (a wavelike motion). The bladder, a sac-like organ made of elastic muscle, stores urine that has flowed through the ureters. When the bladder becomes full of urine, signals indicating the need to urinate are sent to the brain via nerves, allowing urine to flow from the bladder to the urethra. In males, the urethra is approximately 20 cm long, while in females, it is about 4 cm long.

sac-like　袋のような
elastic　弾性のある

via　〜経由で

Note

　泌尿器系は，身体にとって不要なものを体外に排出する器官系です。血液をろ過して作られた尿を体外へ導く尿道には男女差があり，これは生殖器の違いによるものです。男性の尿道は，長く，屈曲していますが，女性の尿道は，短く，ほぼまっすぐ外陰部に続いています。そのため，細菌が侵入して膀胱炎を起こしやすいです。

Point　分詞構文

主語＋動詞，〜ingの文では，〜ing以降の部分で接続詞と主語が省略されており，「そして〜する」と訳します。

例1： He entered the classroom, turning on the light.
　　　彼は教室に入って，（そして）電気をつけた。

例2： The pathway through which urine passes is called the urinary tract, extending from the ureters to the bladder and urethra.
　　　尿が通過する道は尿路と呼ばれ，（そして，）尿管から膀胱を経て尿道へと伸びている。

Drill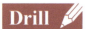

次の英文の1と2は [   ] 内の語句を並び替えて日本語訳に合う英文にし，3と4は日本語訳に合うように空欄に正しい英語を書きなさい。

1. The blood [each glomerulus / exits / through a large renal vein / through finer veins / , ultimately leaving].
   血液は各糸球体をさらに細い静脈を通って出て行き，最終的に，大きな腎静脈を通って流れ出る。
   _____

2. ...signals indicating the need to urinate [, allowing / are sent / to flow / to the brain via nerves / urine] from the bladder to the urethra.
   排尿の必要性を示す信号が神経経由で脳に送られ，そして，尿が膀胱から尿道へ流れることになる。
   _____

3. A Tsunami hit Tohoku area, (   ) huge damage.
   津波は東北地方に上陸し，甚大な被害をもたらした。
   _____

4. He has found Japanese literature interesting, (   ) his research about it.
   彼は日本文学に興味を持ち，それについて研究を始めた。
   _____

Summary

1～6に入る適切な語句を選択肢から選び，本文の要約を完成させなさい。

　泌尿器系は，2つの1)_____と2)_____，膀胱と尿道で構成されており，身体にとって不要となった3)_____を体外に排泄するための器官系である。それぞれの1)_____には約100万個の4)_____と呼ばれる最小の構造物があり，ボーマン嚢と糸球体，尿細管がある。1)_____の主な機能は，体の状態や水と塩分の出入りに合わせて，5)_____の量と成分を調節し，体内の環境を一定に保つことである。2)_____の上端は1)_____に，下端は膀胱につながっており，5)_____は6)_____によってこの2)_____を通って少量ずつ膀胱に送られていく。そして，膀胱がいっぱいになると排尿が必要である信号が脳に送られ，尿道へと流れ出る。

| 選択肢： | 老廃物 | 腎臓 | 尿管 | 尿 | ネフロン | 蠕動運動 |

Questions and Answers QA

本文を読み，次の問に英語で答えなさい。

1. What is the urinary system composed of?

2. Where are the kidneys located?

3. How do nephrons work?

4. How is urine transported to the bladder?

5. What is the difference between the male and female urethra?

Activity

1. 尿を作る腎臓の働きについて，尿ができる仕組みとともに調べてみましょう。
2. 腎臓の働きが悪くなることで発症するかもしれない病気について調べてみましょう。

1.

2.

Chapter 5 The Urinary System **41**

Chapter 6
The Skeletal System
(Bones, joints, and ligaments)

骨格系について学びます。
骨は人体を支え，関節は体を動かすために重要な役割があり，さらに骨に付随する靱帯もあります。

Introduction

次の骨の画像は身体のどの部位ですか？　日本語と英語で答えなさい。

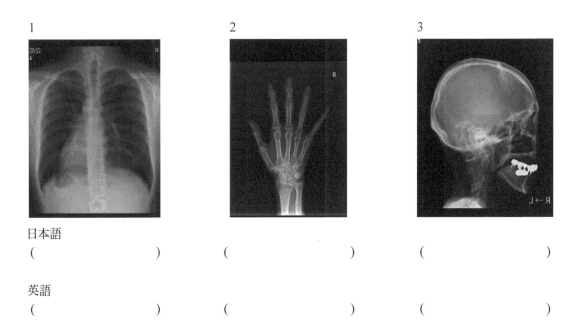

日本語
(　　　　　　　)　　(　　　　　　　　　)　　(　　　　　　　　　)

英語
(　　　　　　　)　　(　　　　　　　　　)　　(　　　　　　　　　)

6-1. Dialogue

大学の食堂で Yoko（Y）と Mari（M）が話しています。

Y: Long time, no see! What happened to your hand? You have a cast on.

M: Yeah, it's been a while since we don't see each other so often now that our campuses are different from last year. Last month, I actually fell down the stairs at home and broke my hand.

Y: What? Ouch! How did you fall?

M: I was carrying some stuff down the stairs, not really looking where I was going, and I missed the third step from the bottom. When I fell, I landed on my right hand and heard a "pop". It hurt a bit, but I just put a cold pack on and came to the university.

Y: Wow, no way! Were you okay coming back to the university like that?

M: The pain got worse after I arrived, so later I went to the health center. The doctor there suspected a fracture and referred me to a nearby clinic for an X-ray. Turns out, I had a broken wrist.

Y: That sounds awful! I can't imagine breaking my wrist like that.

M: The doctor explained that when you fell and landed on your palm, the broken part of the bone shifted towards the back of the hand. This type of fracture is called a Colles' fracture. They gave me painkillers, and I went home. The next day at the clinic, I had surgery to set the bone with a plate, and they put on a cast. Apparently, if you leave a fracture untreated, the bone can heal incorrectly or cause functional problems. I'm glad I got it treated quickly.

Y: Quick treatment is crucial. Do you have to keep the plate in forever?

Long time, no see!
しばらくぶりです

cast　ギプス

where I was going
行先

worse　←bad の比較級

health center
医療施設

fracture　骨折

refer　述べる

turn out　判明する

broken wrist　手首の骨折

shift　位置を変える

leave a fracture untreated
骨折を治療しないままに
しておく

M: No, once the bone is properly healed, they'll perform a second surgery to remove the plate. Then, I'll have the cast removed and after that, start rehabilitation.

Y: That sounds tough. I guess you need rehabilitation because the body loses functionality if you don't move it for a while. Make sure to hold onto the handrails when using stairs from now on, even at the station. I almost fell at the station once when my pants got caught on my heel. Now I always use the handrails. Take care!

M: Thanks! Let's both be careful.

Point 💡 leave ＋ 目的語 ＋ 過去分詞

leave ＋ 目的語 ＋ 過去分詞：〜をそのままにしておく
目的語と動詞の関係が受動態の時，動詞は過去分詞になる。
能動態の時，動詞は現在分詞（~ing）になる。

例：Don't leave a fracture untreated.
　　骨折を治療しないままにしてはいけない。

Drill

以下の文を英語または日本語に訳しなさい。

1. Tom left the door unlocked.
　_____

2. That boy left the water running.
　_____

3. あの子供たちはおもちゃを散らかしたままにした。　（散らかす＝scatter）
　_____

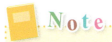

コレス骨折

手のひらをついて転んだり，自転車やバイクに乗っていて転んだりしたときに，前腕の2本の骨のうちの橈骨が手首のところ（遠位端）で折れる骨折。

Questions and Answers

会話文を読み，次の問に英語で答えなさい。

1. How did Mari fall down the stairs?
   _____

2. Why did Mari go to the clinic?
   _____

3. What did the doctor who examined Mari explain about the fracture to her?
   _____

4. Did Mari get surgery?
   _____

5. What can occur if the fracture is left untreated?
   _____

6-2. Reading

Vocabulary

biaxial joint	二軸性関節	multiaxial joint	多軸性関節
bone marrow (hematopoiesis)	骨髄	patella	膝蓋骨
capsular ligament	関節包靭帯	patellar ligament	膝蓋靭帯
carpal bone	手根骨	pneumatic bone	含気骨
cartilage plate	軟骨板	predominantly	主に
compound joint	複合関節	scapula	肩甲骨
cylindrical bone	円筒形の骨	sesamoid bone	種子骨
endochondral ossification	軟骨内骨化	short bone	短骨
extracapsular ligament	関節包外靭帯	simple joint	単関節
femur	大腿骨	skull	頭蓋骨
flat bone	扁平骨	sphenoid	蝶形骨
humerus	上腕骨	spongy bone	海綿骨
iliac bone	腸骨	stabilizing	安定化作用
irregular bone	不規則骨	sternoclavicular joint	胸鎖関節
joint cavity	関節腔	synovial fluid	滑液
ligament	靭帯	synovial membrane	滑膜
limb	四肢	tarsal bone	足根骨
long (tubular) bone	長骨	tendon	腱
maxilla	上顎骨	uniaxial joint	一軸性関節
membranous ossification	膜性骨化	vertebra	椎骨

Bones

    Bones are very hard tissues composed of fibers and minerals. They serve several important functions, such as maintaining body shape, protecting internal organs, producing blood in the bone marrow (hematopoiesis), and storing minerals. There are 206 bones in the human body, classified as follows:

be composed of〜
〜で構成されている

such as　〜のような

as follows　次のように

1. Long (Tubular) Bones: These are long, cylindrical bones with expanded ends (e.g., humerus, femur).
2. Short Bones: These are small, short bones predominantly made up of spongy bone (e.g., carpal bones, tarsal bones).
3. Flat Bones: These are flat bones consisting of a spongy bone layer sandwiched between two layers of compact bone (e.g., skull bones, iliac bones).
4. Irregular Bones: These bones have complex shapes with various features (e.g., scapula, vertebra).
5. Pneumatic Bones: These bones contain air-filled cavities (e.g., maxilla, sphenoid).

Small, similarly shaped, rounded bones that develop within ligaments or tendons are called sesamoid bones. The largest sesamoid bone is the patella, located within the patellar ligament.

Bone Growth

Bone growth occurs through two processes: membranous ossification and endochondral ossification. The former involves the formation of bone from a membrane, as seen in the skull and iliac bones, while the latter involves the ossification of growth cartilage plates, as seen in the femur and humerus. Typically, bone growth continues until about ages 17-18 in males and 15-16 in females.

Joints

A joint is a structure formed by the connection of two or more bones, linking the skeletal system and facilitating its overall function. Joints are classified based on the number of bones involved and their movement. A joint formed by two bones is called a simple joint, while one formed by three or more bones is called a compound joint. Joints are also classified by their movement: uniaxial joints move around a single axis, biaxial joints move around two perpendicular axes, and multiaxial joints move in multiple directions around three or more axes. Furthermore, joints are classified as either movable (synovial) or immovable. Most joints in the limbs are movable joints, where the inner surface of the joint is covered by synovial membranes and synovial fluid is found in the joint cavity, hence being called "synovial joints". Immovable joints lack synovial membranes, joint cavities, and synovial fluid. Instead, these joints have connective tissue between the bones, as seen in the sternoclavicular joint.

Joints are also categorized by their shape, including ball-and-socket joints, saddle joints, pivot joints, ellipsoidal joints, hinge joints, and plane joints.

instead 代わりに

be categorized by ～によって分類される

Ligaments

Ligaments are crucial components of joints, connecting bones to bones. Their functions include stabilizing the joints and limiting the range of motion. Capsular ligaments enhance the strength of the joint capsule, while extracapsular ligaments prevent bone separation and improve joint stability.

, connecting ～を連結する

while 一方

Point 💡 分詞の後置修飾

分詞が前の名詞を修飾します。(名詞に修飾語がついている場合は後ろから修飾します)
　　hard tissues composed of fibers and minerals～
　　繊維やミネラルで構成されている固い組織
➡ 下線部が前の名詞を修飾します。動詞と名詞の関係が受動態の時, 動詞は過去分詞になります。
　　short bones made up of ～
　　～でつくられている短骨
　　分詞の後置修飾で前の名詞を修飾します。
　　flat bones consisting of ～
　　～で構成されている扁平骨

Drill ✏️

( ) 内の動詞を適切な形にしなさい。

1. Look at the baby (cry) in the bed there.

2. I found my key (lose) in the car yesterday.

3. He repaired the (break) chair today.

48

Questions and Answers

本文を読み，次の問に英語で答えなさい。

1. What are the bones made up of?
   _____

2. What functions do bones have?
   _____

3. How many bones are in the body?
   _____

4. What is the biggest sesamoid bone in the human body?
   _____

5. How are joints classified?
   _____

6. What functions do ligaments have?
   _____

Summary

1～10に入る適切な語句を選択肢から選び，本文の要約を完成させなさい。

　骨は，線維とミネラルからなる非常に硬い組織である。骨には，「体形を保持する」「内臓を保護する」「骨髄で血液を造る（造血）」「1) _____」などの重要な機能がある。
　骨の成長は，2) _____ と軟骨内骨化による。前者は，頭蓋骨，腸骨などのような3) _____ による骨形成であり，後者は，大腿骨，上腕骨などのような4) _____ の骨化により骨の成長が起こる。これらの骨は一般的に男性では5) _____ くらい，女性では6) _____ くらいまで成長する。相対する2つまたはそれ以上の骨で連結された構造体が7) _____ と呼ばれ，これらの関節が骨格系と骨格の機能全体とを関連づけている。構成する骨の数と8) _____ により分類されている。2個の骨で形成されるものは9) _____，3個以上の骨で形成されるものは10) _____ と呼ばれる。

選択肢：	膜性骨化	ミネラルを貯蔵する		単関節	動き	成長軟骨板
	17～18歳	関節	15～16歳	骨膜	複合関節	

Chapter 6 The Skeletal System (Bones, joints, ligaments)　**49**

Activity

（1）空欄に骨の種類を日本語と英語で記入しましょう。

	日本語	英語
長骨		
短骨		
扁平骨		
不規則骨		
含気骨		

(2) それぞれの骨の名前を日本語と英語で調べましょう。

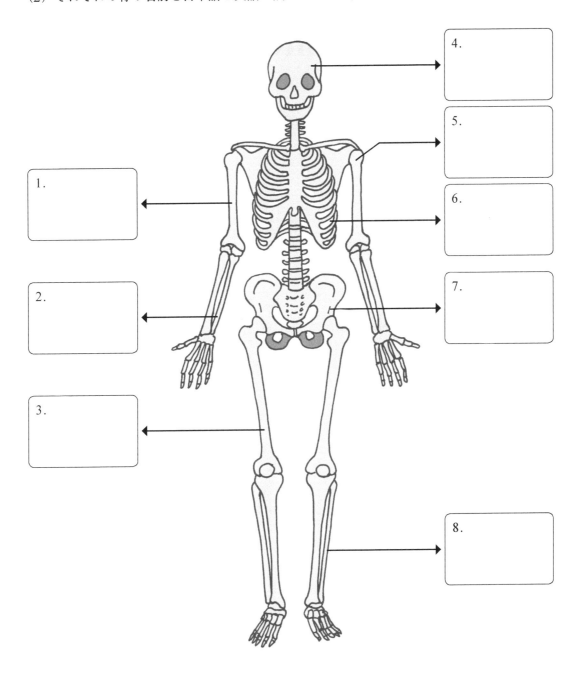

1.
2.
3.
4.
5.
6.
7.
8.

Chapter 6 The Skeletal System (Bones, joints, ligaments) **51**

Chapter 7

Food-Drug Interactions

薬と食品の飲み合わせについて学びます。

Introduction

以下は食品と薬の飲み合わせによる相互作用を示す図です。1〜6に入る語句を選択肢から選んで空欄に記入しましょう。

含まれる成分		及ぼす影響
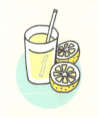 (1)	+ →	(4)
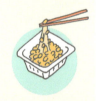 (2)	+ 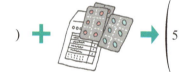 →	(5)
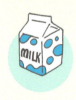 (3)	+ →	(6)

選択肢:
furanocoumarin   higher-than-normal concentration of the drug in the blood
vitamin K   weaken the effects of anticoagulants
calcium   hinder absorption in the body

7-1. Dialogue

薬局でMs. Mori（M）が，薬剤師のMs. Ito（I）に服用している薬と食品の飲み合わせについて尋ねています。

M: Hello. I am currently taking medication for high blood pressure. Recently, I've been drinking a lot of grapefruit juice because it's rich in vitamin C and good for my health. However, I am concerned about whether it's safe to drink it while taking this medication.

I: I see. There is, in fact, an interaction between grapefruit and high blood pressure medication. The furanocoumarins found in grapefruit can inhibit drug-metabolizing enzymes, which may affect how the medication works and cause side effects.

M: Is my medication okay?

I: Actually, since you are taking calcium antagonists for your high blood pressure, you need to be cautious about combining them with grapefruit. This combination can increase the drug's concentration in your blood, potentially causing symptoms of low blood pressure.

M: I see, what a surprise! I didn't realize how important it is to know the relationship between food and medication. How can I be more careful in the future?

I: It is best to either avoid drinking grapefruit juice with your medication altogether, or simply adjust the timing of when you take your medication. In the future, if you need specific instructions regarding your medication, it would be good to consult with your doctor or pharmacist in advance.

M: Got it. Thank you very much.

---

high blood pressure
高血圧

be rich in　〜が豊富である

be good for
（健康・身体など）に良い

be concerned about
〜について心配している

interaction　相互作用

furanocoumarin
フラノクマリン

drug-metabolizing enzyme
薬物代謝酵素

calcium antagonist
カルシウム拮抗薬

either A or B
AかBのどちらか

regarding　〜について

consult with
〜と相談する

in advance　事前に

Chapter 7 Food-Drug Interactions　**53**

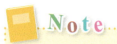

medicine と medication

「薬」の英語はmedicineと思い浮かびますが，ここではmedicationが使われています。medicineは，一般的に「薬」や「医学」を指し，市販薬・処方薬など広範囲を含みます。一方，medicationは，「薬の服用」や「投薬治療」の意味が強く，特に医師の指示に基づく処方薬を指すことが多いです。

Point 仮主語と真主語

it is important to~ は，「～することは大切だ」という表現です。英語では長い主語を嫌いますから，it（仮主語）で置き換えて本当の主語（真主語）はto以下で示します。

例1：It is important to know the relationship between food and medication.
　　　食べ物と薬の関係を知ることは，大切だ。

例2：It is okay to drink it while taking this medication.
　　　この薬を服用している間にそれを飲んでも大丈夫だ。

Drill

空欄に入る適切な語句を選択肢から選び，記号で書きなさい。

1. Working out regularly is (　　　) for you.

2. They will discuss various environmental issues, (　　　), climate change.

3. This soil is (　　　) in minerals for plants to grow.

4. You should tell your teacher about it (　　　).

5. I am (　　　) about my father in hospital.

| (a) concerned | (b) in specific | (c) rich |
| (d) in advance | (e) good | |

Questions and Answers Q&A

会話文を読み，次の問に英語で答えなさい。

1. What is Ms. Mori concerned about?

2. What advice does the pharmacist give about taking medication for high blood pressure?

7-2. Reading

Vocabulary

antagonist	拮抗薬	furanocoumarin	フラノクマリン
antibiotics	抗生物質	medication	投薬, 薬剤
anticoagulant	抗凝固剤	metabolize	代謝する
antihypertensive	抗高血圧性の	side effect	副作用
calcium	カルシウム	thrombosis	血栓症
enzyme	酵素	vitamin K	ビタミンK

There are certain combinations of medication and food that do not mix well. Consuming certain foods after taking the medication can influence its action, such as enhancing or diminishing its effectiveness and causing side effects that may harm your health. For example, grapefruit juice contains furanocoumarins, which have the property of inhibiting drug-metabolizing enzymes. This makes it harder for antihypertensive drugs (for example, calcium antagonists), absorbed from the small intestine, to be metabolized by these enzymes, resulting in a higher-than-normal concentration of the drug in the blood. When this kind of combination occurs, excessive amounts of the drug can remain in the system, causing blood pressure to drop excessively, or other strong side effects. It is not uncommon for drugs to interact with components in food like this.

On the other hand, other foods and beverages can affect the efficacy of medications. For example, foods high in vitamin K (such as

enhance　強める

diminish　減らす, 弱める

harm　害を及ぼす

property　特性

inhibit　抑止する

excessively　過度に

interact with〜
〜と相互作用する

on the other hand　一方

efficacy　効き目・効用

Chapter 7 Food-Drug Interactions　**55**

natto and spinach) are known to weaken the effects of anticoagulants used for treating thrombosis. Natto contains natto bacteria that produce vitamin K in the body, which in turn reduces the effectiveness of anticoagulants. Moreover, dairy products like milk and cheese can interfere with the absorption of certain antibiotics. Milk contains a high amount of calcium, which can bind with components of specific antibiotics, hindering their absorption in the body. Consequently, taking these foods together with antibiotics can prevent the medication from working effectively. It is important to be cautious, as your choice of food and drink can significantly impact the effectiveness and safety of medications.

in turn 次に, 順番に

interfere with
〜に干渉する, 〜を妨げる

bind with〜
〜と結合する

hinder 妨げる

prevent ... from〜
…が〜するのを防ぐ

Pharmacists play a crucial role in providing information about the relationship between food and the medications that patients are taking. To ensure that patients take their medications safely, pharmacists must have a strong knowledge of drug-food interactions and provide appropriate advice. Furthermore, pharmacists need to consider the patient's lifestyle and eating habits, offering tailored advice accordingly. For instance, if avoiding certain foods is difficult, it may be necessary to suggest alternatives. To help patients take their medications with confidence, pharmacists should continuously gather the latest information and provide accurate, up-to-date guidance.

play a role in〜
〜において役割をはたす

crucial 重要な

tailored 適合した

alternative 代替品

up-to-date 最新の

Point 💡 接続副詞

前の文と後ろの文を結ぶ接続詞のような働きをする副詞が, 本文中によく見られます。接続副詞といわれるものですが, いろいろな意味を表します。

1. for example, for instance 「例えば,」と例を挙げる。
2. on the other hand 「一方で,」と反対のことを述べる。
3. moreover, furthermore 「さらに,」と追加する。
4. consequently 「よって,」「したがって,」と結論を述べる。

Drill

空欄に入る適切な語句を選択肢から選び，記号で書きなさい。文頭に来るものも小文字になっています。

1. He didn't study the right book. (　　), he failed his exams.

2. This jacket is a little bit small. (　　), the style has become out of fashion.

3. I recommend you eat some fruits every morning, (　　), kiwi and banana.

4. My elder brother likes pork curry. (　　) my younger brother likes beef curry.

5. He works so hard. (　　), he often stays late at this office and coaches the children's baseball team every weekend.

(a) consequently	(b) furthermore	(c) in fact
(d) for example	(e) on the other hand	

Summary

1～6に入る適切な語句を選択肢から選び，本文の要約を完成させなさい。

　　グレープフルーツジュースには，フラノクマリンという1)＿＿＿＿＿を阻害する成分が含まれており，薬の服用時には，場合によっては，過剰な薬物効果が現れ，2)＿＿＿＿＿が強く出る可能性がある。また，納豆菌によって体内で生成されるビタミンKは，血栓治療に使用される3)＿＿＿＿＿の効果を減弱したり，牛乳中のカルシウムは，特定の4)＿＿＿＿＿の成分と結合することで，その体内吸収を阻害したりする。よって，薬の服用時には5)＿＿＿＿＿や飲み物の選択に注意が必要である。薬の専門家として6)＿＿＿＿＿は，患者が安全に薬を服用できるように，薬と食品の相互作用について，個別に適切なアドバイスを提供する。

| 選択肢： | 抗凝固剤 | 抗生物質 | 食事 | 副作用 | 薬剤師 | 薬物代謝酵素 |

Questions and Answers QA

本文を読み，次の問に英語で答えなさい。

1. What are the properties of grapefruit juice?

2. What does vitamin K do in the body?

3. Why is it important to be cautious about food and drink choices when taking medication?

4. What do pharmacists play a crucial role in?

5. What should pharmacists do to help patients be confident when taking their medications?

Activity

本文以外に薬と食品の組み合わせで気を付けるべき例を調べてみましょう。

食養生と_____「薬膳」を学びます。「薬膳」は薬が多く入れられた食事ではなく_____のことです。

Introdu...

薬膳の例

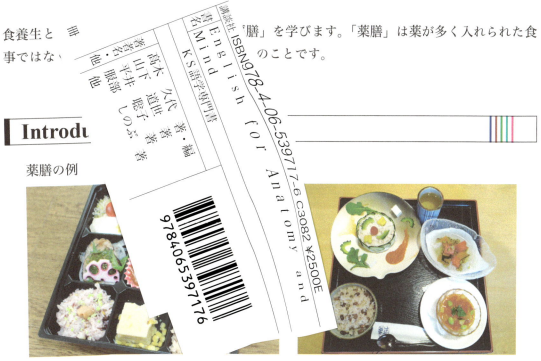

薬膳は昔から食養生として知られています。食材は体を冷やすもの，体を温めるものに分けられます。下記から適切なものを選び（　　）を埋めましょう。

1. 体を温める食材（　　　　　）（　　　　　　）（　　　　　　）

2. 体を冷やす食材（　　　　　）（　　　　　　）（　　　　　　）

キュウリ　　カボチャ　　エビ　　トマト　　ゴーヤ　　シナモン

Chapter 8　Yakuzen　59

8-1. Dialogue

最近薬膳がより一般的になっていますが，どのような料理が薬膳であるのか理解していない人が多いようです。栄養学科のMay（M）が高校時代の友人Yukari（Y）と話しています。

Y: Recently, I've seen the term "yakuzen" a lot in magazines. Is it a type of Chinese cuisine?

M: Many people think that, but yakuzen is about "dietary therapy." It's a way of thinking about meals as a way to care for your body. Japanese cuisine, French cuisine, or any cuisine can be yakuzen.

dietary therapy
食事療法, 食養生

Y: There's an English saying, "You are what you eat." Does this also mean "yakuzen"?

what you eat
あなたが食べたもの

M: There's also an old Chinese saying, "Life is in food." This idea that is a connection between life and food, is found in both Eastern and Western cultures. We are made of what we eat, thus we need to pay attention to what we eat every day.

Life is in food
命は食にあり

pay attention to
〜に注意をする

Y: Meals are a part of our health that we can control, but when you go to the store, they sell all sorts of things, so it's hard to know what's good for us.

it is hard to know
〜を知るのは難しい

M: I'm currently studying yakuzen at university. Let me explain a bit.

Y: Wow, you study yakuzen in addition to nutrition at university?

in addition to
〜に加えて

nutrition　栄養

M: Yes. Studying both nutrition and yakuzen allows us to create more appropriate meals for people. Some people think yakuzen involves food with medicine in it, but it's actually about meals that make the body healthy like medicine does. It's about choosing foodstuffs that match the season, local area, and condition of the person eating them. Essentially, when making meals, we should use seasonal foodstuffs, local foodstuffs, and foodstuffs

make the body healthy
体を健康にさせる

60

Chapter 8

Yakuzen

食養生として中国医学を背景にした「薬膳」を学びます。「薬膳」は薬が多く入れられた食事ではなく，体に良く美味しい食事（膳）のことです。

Introduction

薬膳の例

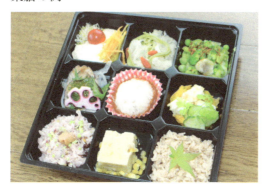 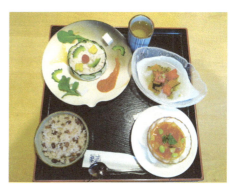

薬膳は昔から食養生として知られています。食材は体を冷やすもの，体を温めるものに分けられます。下記から適切なものを選び（　　）を埋めましょう。

1. 体を温める食材（　　　　　　）（　　　　　　）（　　　　　　）

2. 体を冷やす食材（　　　　　　）（　　　　　　）（　　　　　　）

キュウリ　　カボチャ　　エビ　　トマト　　ゴーヤ　　シナモン

8-1. Dialogue

最近薬膳がより一般的になっていますが，どのような料理が薬膳であるのか理解していない人が多いようです。栄養学科のMay（M）が高校時代の友人Yukari（Y）と話しています。

Y: Recently, I've seen the term "yakuzen" a lot in magazines. Is it a type of Chinese cuisine?

M: Many people think that, but yakuzen is about "dietary therapy." It's a way of thinking about meals as a way to care for your body. Japanese cuisine, French cuisine, or any cuisine can be yakuzen.

> dietary therapy
> 食事療法, 食養生

Y: There's an English saying, "You are what you eat." Does this also mean "yakuzen"?

> what you eat
> あなたが食べたもの

M: There's also an old Chinese saying, "Life is in food." This idea that is a connection between life and food, is found in both Eastern and Western cultures. We are made of what we eat, thus we need to pay attention to what we eat every day.

> Life is in food
> 命は食にあり

> pay attention to
> 〜に注意をする

Y: Meals are a part of our health that we can control, but when you go to the store, they sell all sorts of things, so it's hard to know what's good for us.

> it is hard to know
> 〜を知るのは難しい

M: I'm currently studying yakuzen at university. Let me explain a bit.

Y: Wow, you study yakuzen in addition to nutrition at university?

> in addition to
> 〜に加えて

> nutrition　栄養

M: Yes. Studying both nutrition and yakuzen allows us to create more appropriate meals for people. Some people think yakuzen involves food with medicine in it, but it's actually about meals that make the body healthy like medicine does. It's about choosing foodstuffs that match the season, local area, and condition of the person eating them. Essentially, when making meals, we should use seasonal foodstuffs, local foodstuffs, and foodstuffs

> make the body healthy
> 体を健康にさせる

that suit our health condition.

Y: I often hear that seasonal food is good. Does that mean we should avoid eating summer vegetables like cucumbers, eggplants, and bitter melons in winter?

cucumber　キュウリ

eggplant　ナス

bitter melon　ゴーヤ

M: That's right. Summer vegetables have a cooling effect on the body, so it's better not to eat them too much in winter. For example, tomatoes are good for you because they contain lycopene, but they also have a cooling effect. Therefore, it's better not to enjoy them in the middle of winter.

therefore　それ故に

Y: I didn't know some foodstuffs have a cooling effect on the body! I'm getting interested in yakuzen. I want to study it too.

M: I have some books, so let's study together. It'll be fun!

Point 💡 関係代名詞のwhat，仮主語のit，使役動詞のmake

関係代名詞のwhat：先行詞を含む関係代名詞，something which のことです。

You are <u>what</u> you eat.

あなた達は自分で食べたものでできている

➡ 下線部 what は先行詞を含む関係代名詞　〜のこと，〜のもの

仮主語のit：it は仮主語で，to 以下が本当の主語です。

It is hard to know.

知ることは難しい。

使役動詞のmake：〜を〜させる

Yakuzen <u>makes</u> the body healthy just like medicine does.

薬膳は薬と同じように体を健康にする。

Chapter 8 Yakuzen　**61**

Drill

以下の文章を日本語に訳しなさい。

1. It is important for medical students to study anatomy and physiology.
   _____

2. It is difficult for me to speak and write English.
   _____

Questions and Answers

会話文を読み，次の問に英語で答えなさい。

1. What is yakuzen?
   _____

2. What effects do summer foodstuffs have on the body?
   _____

8-2. Reading

Vocabulary

broth	薄い澄んだスープ	root vegetable	根野菜
counteract	和らげる, 中和する	*shindo fuji*	身土不二
detoxify	解毒する, 無毒にする	*shinshin ichinyo*	心身一如（心も体も結びついているという考え）
disturbance	乱すこと, 動揺, 不安	tailor	合わせる
Huangdi Neijing	黄帝内経（中国最古の医書）	traditional Japanese cuisine	伝統日本料理（和食）
kelp	海藻		

Considering Food in Oriental Medicine

The ancient Chinese medical text known as the *Huangdi Neijing*, or "The Yellow Emperor's Classic of Internal Medicine," has been regarded as the bible of Oriental Medicine for over 2,000 years. It reads, "Life is in food. If food is incorrect, illness occurs; if food is correct, illness naturally heals." The English proverb "You are what you eat" similarly reflects this universal truth about the relationship between food and health. Another key concept in Oriental Medicine is *shinshin ichinyo*, which means "the mind and body are one," indicating that mental disturbances affect the body, and physical disturbances affect the mind. Thus, healthy food is fundamental to cultivating a healthy body and mind.

Nowadays, with more people paying attention to their diet, there is growing interest in "medicinal cuisine" or yakuzen, which has long been practiced in China as "dietary therapy." Here are the basic principles of yakuzen.

Three Guidelines for Adaptation:

1. Adaptation to Time: Use seasonal ingredients.
   Seasonal foods come to their nutritional peak during their respective seasons and contain the nutrients necessary for that time of year. For example, in winter, root vegetables like radish and cabbage warm the body, while in summer, ingredients like bitter melon, cucumbers, and tomatoes cool the body.

2. Adaptation to Place: Use locally sourced ingredients.
   There is a saying, *shindo fuji*, which means "the body and the land are inseparable." This means consuming locally grown foods while they are in season ensures the body will receive the nutrients it needs for that time of year.

3. Adaptation to the Individual: Eat foods suited to the individual's constitution which refer to one's personal condition, their body type, age, sex, and health condition.
   Instead of taking medicine when feeling unwell, one should eat meals that are gentle on the stomach and tailored to their physical condition to regain strength.

have been regarded as
〜として考えられている，
〜としてみなされている

concept 概念

mental disturbances
心の不調

medicinal cuisine 薬膳

has long been practiced
ずっと実践されてきた

Adaptation to Time
いん じ せい ぎ
因時制宜

Adaptation to Place
いん ち せい ぎ
因地制宜

Adaptation to the Individual
いんじんせい ぎ
因人制宜

instead of 〜の代わりに

Chapter 8 Yakuzen **63**

In addition to these three principles of yakuzen, traditional Japanese cuisine, or "*washoku*," and its seasoning methods are also important.

Washoku

The traditional "one soup, three dishes" format of washoku was designed with nutritional balance in mind. The principles underlying yakuzen were introduced to Japan by Japanese envoys to Tang China and thus incorporated into washoku. These yakuzen principles are present in pairings such as tempura with grated radish (which aids digestion), sashimi with shiso and wasabi (which have detoxifying properties and warm the body) and soba with green onions and shichimi, or "seven-spice powder" (which counteract the cooling effect of the noodles on the body).

Seasoning

Washoku utilizes a broth called *dashi*, made from bonito, kelp, and shiitake mushrooms. This dashi contains umami components that enhance the natural flavors of ingredients and make it easier to fully appreciate the taste of food. Should you only consume strongly flavored dishes, your palate can dull over time. However, washoku tends to contain more salt compared to Western cuisine, so it's important to be mindful of your salt intake.

We hope that you will continue your "journey to eat your way to maintaining a healthy lifestyle" by enjoying delicious meals suited to your needs.

in addition to	〜に加えて
grated	すり下ろした
detoxifying properties	解毒する成分
a broth called *dashi*,	だしと呼ばれる汁
natural flavors	自然の風味
make it easier to	〜するのをより簡単にする
be mindful of	〜を意識している

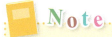

『黄帝内経（*Huangdi Neijing*）』は中国最古の医書。中国医学のバイブルと呼ばれている。黄帝に仮託した，戦国時代から漢にかけての医学知識の結集。18巻で〈素問〉と〈霊枢〉からなる。

（百科事典マイペディアより）

Point 現在完了の受動態

現在完了の受動態：have (has) ＋ been（be動詞の過去分詞）＋ 過去分詞
　過去の時点から今現在まで〜されている，〜された，〜されたことがある

　　has been regarded as　〜として考えられている／〜としてみなされている
　　has long been practiced　ずっと実践されている（されてきた）

Drill

以下の文章を日本語に訳しなさい。

1. Practicing makes it easier for acupuncturists to examine patients.
　_____

2. Staying indoors too often makes it harder for elderly people to move by themselves.
　_____

Questions and Answers

本文を読み，次の問に英語で答えなさい。

1. What is the *Huangdi Neijing*?
　_____

2. What does the phrase *Shindo Fuji* mean?
　_____

3. Explain about Adaptation to Time.
　_____

4. Explain about Adaptation to the Individual.
　_____

5. What is dashi?
　_____

6. What was introduced to Japan by Japanese envoys to Tang China?
　_____

Summary 📄

1〜6に入る適切な語句を選択肢から選び，本文の要約を完成させなさい。

　　はるか2000年以上前から伝えられ東洋医学のバイブルといわれる古典1) ＿＿＿＿＿＿ には，「**命は食にあり，食誤れば病たり，食正しければ病自ずと癒える**」とある。また東洋医学には2) ＿＿＿＿＿＿ という言葉があり，「心と体は結びついており，心の不調は身体に，身体の不調は心に影響を及ぼす」を意味する。

　　「3) ＿＿＿＿＿＿ 」とは，四季にあった旬の食材を選ぶことである。旬の食材はその時期に栄養価が高く，体の調子を整えてくれる。例えば，冬には体を中から温める根野菜の大根，白菜が，夏には体を冷やしてくれるゴーヤ，キュウリ，トマト等がある。

　　人間の体とその人が住む土地は切り離すことができず，それを表す「4) ＿＿＿＿＿＿ 」という言葉がある。人はその人が住む土地に応じた，その土地に合ったものを食べる。これを5) ＿＿＿＿＿＿ という。また，その土地でできた食材を使用することを地産地消という。

　　体質，年齢，性別，体調に合ったものを食べる「6) ＿＿＿＿＿＿ 」という言葉がある。体調が悪い時に薬を飲むのではなく，体調，体質に合わせ胃に優しい食事をすることで体力を回復させることができる。

選択肢： 身土不二　　　黄帝内経　　　因人制宜　　　因地制宜　　　因時制宜　　　心身一如

Activity

日本でよく使用される生薬の効能を調べましょう。写真は何の生薬ですか？ グループで調べましょう。

緑豆　　　　ナツメ　　　ショウガ　　　竜眼　　　ハスの実　　　クコ

	生薬の名前	生薬の効能
1		
2		
3		
4		
5		
6		

Chapter 8　Yakuzen　**67**

Chapter 9

Stress

日々のストレスが心身にどのような影響を与えるかを考え，上手に付き合うコツを学びます。

Introduction

あなたはどんな時にストレスを感じますか？
ストレスを感じると心身にどのような変化が
起こりますか？

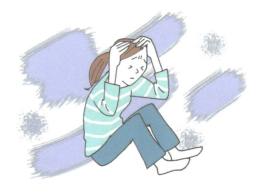

どんな時にストレスを感じますか？　具体的に書き出してみましょう。

ストレスを感じる時，心や体調にどのような変化が起こりますか？

9-1. Dialogue

Riku（R）と Megu（M）が学食で話していると，担当教員の Mr. Nakanishi（N）とばったり出会い，話し始めます。

R: Class lasts until 12:40 but I get dizzy when I'm hungry.

lasts until 〜まで続く

M: Lately, I've been tired and don't have much of an appetite.

appetite 食欲

N (Professor): Come to think of it, have you been losing weight?

come to think of it そういえば

M: Actually, yeah. It might be because when I have reports due, I sometimes skip dinner.

N: That's not good. You might be accumulating stress from having so many report submissions and exams. Many people in Japan today are under stress due to being too busy or dealing with interpersonal issues. Signs of stress include irritability, loss of appetite, and fatigue. It would be wise to find a healthy way to relieve your stress.

accumulating stress ストレスを溜める

deal with〜 〜に対処する

irritability イライラ

fatigue 疲労

R: Yeah, university students deal with a lot of stress. What should we do to unwind?

unwind リラックスする

N: I suggest you make time to hang with your friends. When I'm busy and feeling irritable, I make sure to talk to my friends instead of bottling it up. You could also go somewhere to refresh yourself. I sometimes go to the movie theater to relax and unwind.

hang with your friends 友達と過ごす

bottling it up 抱え込む

M: It's important not to bottle things up, isn't it? Although, we also shouldn't let report writing pile up.

pile up 溜まる

N: If you ever need someone to talk to, come by my office. We can talk about anything on your mind over coffee.

R, M: Thank you, professor!

Chapter 9 Stress **69**

Point 💡 instead of ~ing

instead of ~ingは，何かをする代わりに別の行動をとる場合に使います。この時，instead ofの後に動名詞を使ってその行動を表現します。

例1：He went to the gym instead of sleeping all day.
　　　彼は一日中寝る代わりにジムに行った。

例2：I decided to eat a salad instead of eating fast food.
　　　私はファストフードを食べる代わりにサラダを食べることにした。

Drill ✐

次の英文の［　　］内の語句を並び替えて，日本語訳に合う英文にしなさい。

1. The meeting ［ the project / until / is / discussed / lasts ］.
　　会議はプロジェクトが議論されるまで続く。

　　_____

2. Come to ［ it / I / , / think / drink / of / should ］ more water daily.
　　考えてみると，もっと毎日水を飲むべきだ。

　　_____

3. Accumulating ［ can / your / immune / harm / stress / system ］.
　　ストレスが積み重なると，免疫システムに害を与えることがある。

　　_____

4. It's important ［ early / with / health / mental / to / issues / deal ］.
　　精神的な健康問題には早期に対処することが重要だ。

　　_____

5. She should ［ of / instead / to / keeping / talk / someone ］ her feelings inside.
　　彼女は感情を内に秘めるのではなく，誰かに話すべきだ。

　　_____

Questions and Answers ᑫᴀ

会話文を読み，次の問に英語で答えなさい。

1. What are the three signs of stress mentioned by the professor?

_____

2. Where does the professor go to refresh himself?

_____

3. What drink will the professor give them in his office?

_____

9-2. Reading

According to the Comprehensive Survey of Living Conditions, one out of every two Japanese people reports having worries or stress in their daily lives. In this report, the main causes of stress included "schoolwork, exams, and further education" and "relationships outside the family" for those aged 12-19, while "work" and "income/household finances" were predominant for those aged 20-60. Additionally, people in their 30s to 50s frequently cited "childcare" and "children's education" as stressors, while those over 50 cited "personal illness or caregiving" and "family illness or caregiving". Given that many people experience stress and that its causes are constantly changing, it is crucial to learn how to manage stress effectively rather than trying to eliminate it completely.

Our first tip for managing stress effectively is to recognize the signs of stress early. Common signs of stress include feeling depressed, irritable, or not enjoying the activities that usually bring you joy. Physical signs can include insomnia, a loss of appetite, headaches, fatigue, and gastrointestinal issues such as diarrhea or constipation. By recognizing these signs early and taking appropriate actions—such as taking a break, engaging in activities that lift your spirits, talking to family or friends, or consulting a mental health professional—you can manage stress effectively. Just as with physical health, the early detection and treatment of mental health issues can prevent them from becoming severe.

comprehensive survey 包括的調査

household finances 家計

predominant   支配的な

effectively   効果的に

gastrointestinal   胃腸の

appropriate   適切な

severe   深刻な

Chapter 9 Stress **71**

Our second tip for managing stress effectively is to focus on the "here and now." We exist on a timeline of past, present, and future. While we cannot change the past, dwelling on it and regretting decisions can lead to depressive mood. Conversely, worrying excessively about the future can cause anxiety. A Buddhist scripture, *Bhaddekaratta-sutta*, teaches that not regretting the past, not worrying about the future, and doing your best in the present will improve your psychological well-being. Thinking practically, if your current situation is tough, you might think, "I'm suffering because of past failures," or "Since things are so hard right now, I have no hope for the future." On the other hand, if your current situation improves, you are less likely to be haunted by past failures and more likely to have hope for the future. The teachings of the Buddha found in *Bhaddekaratta-sutta* have been incorporated into modern mental health practices, such as mindfulness-based stress reduction used in mental health training at global companies like Apple and Google. Using such methods, you, too, can enhance your stress management skills and build resilience against stress.

timeline	時間軸
regret	後悔する
depressive	抑うつの
anxiety	不安
Buddhist scripture	仏教経典
Bhaddekaratta-sutta	バッデーカラッタ・スッタ（一夜賢者経）
on the other hand	一方で
incorporated	取り入れられる
resilience	回復力

Point 💡 on the other hand

on the other hand は「一方で」「その反面」といった意味をもち，対比や異なる視点を示すときに使います。ある意見や状況を述べた後，それとは異なる視点や反対の立場を述べるときに便利な表現です。

例 1 ： Eating fast food is convenient. On the other hand, it can be bad for your health.
ファストフードは便利です。一方で，健康には良くないかもしれません。

例 2 ： Exercising regularly keeps you fit. On the other hand, overtraining can lead to injuries.
定期的な運動は体を健康に保ちます。その反面，やりすぎるとケガの原因になります。

Summary

1～5に入る適切な語句を選択肢から選び，本文の要約を完成させなさい。

　日本人の半数が日常生活でストレスを感じており，12～19歳では1) ＿＿＿＿＿，20～60歳では2) ＿＿＿＿＿や「収入」，30～50代は「子育て」，50代以上では3) ＿＿＿＿＿や「介護」が主な要因である。ストレス対策としては，兆候を早めに4) ＿＿＿＿＿し，休息や楽しい活動，専門家への相談を通じて悪化を防ぐことが重要である。また，過去や未来にとらわれず，「今，この瞬間」に5) ＿＿＿＿＿して最善を尽くすことが幸福につながる。

選択肢：	集中	認識	仕事	勉強	病気

Drill

次の英文の［　　　］内の語句を並び替えて，日本語訳に合う英文にしなさい。

1. Stress is ［ affects / predominant / factor / that / a ］ mental health and overall well-being.
　ストレスは，メンタルヘルスや全体的な健康に影響を与える主要な要因である。

_____

2. It is important to ［ way / stress / find / to / manage / an appropriate ］ in daily life.
　日常生活の中でストレスを管理する適切な方法を見つけることが重要である。

_____

3. Taking breaks and getting ［ sleep / help reduce / effectively / stress / enough ］.
　休憩をとることや十分な睡眠をとることは，ストレスを効果的に軽減するのに役立つ。

_____

4. Lack of rest can ［ severe / physical / and / mental / exhaustion / cause ］.
　休息の不足は深刻な精神的・肉体的疲労を引き起こす可能性がある。

_____

5. Some people cope with stress through exercise, ［ others / to / talking / prefer / on the other hand, ］ to a friend or therapist.
　ストレス対策として運動をする人もいれば，一方で友人やセラピストに相談することを好む人もいる。

_____

Chapter 9 Stress

Questions and Answers

本文を読み，次の問に英語で答えなさい。

1. According to the Comprehensive Survey of Living Conditions, how many Japanese people report having worries or stress in their daily lives?

   _____

2. What does *Bhaddekaratta-sutta* teach?

   _____

3. How can you recognize early signs of stress?

   _____

4. Why is it important to focus on the present moment?

   _____

5. What can you do if you feel stressed?

   _____

Activity

以下の英文を参考にして，友人やクラスメートのストレス解消法について英語で質問してみましょう。答える人は，できるだけ具体的に答えるようにしましょう。

質問文の例：

What do you usually do to relieve stress? Can you describe it in detail?
どんな方法でストレスを解消しますか？　具体的に教えてください。

How do you feel after doing something to relax? Can you explain the process?
リラックスすることをした後，どんな気分になりますか？　その過程を説明してください。

回答例：

I like to read books to escape from stress and relax my mind.
私は本を読むことでストレスから逃れ，心をリラックスさせます。

When I'm stressed, I often take a hot bath to help soothe my body and mind.
ストレスを感じたときは，よく熱いお風呂に入って体と心を癒します。

Listening to my favorite music helps me calm down and forget about my worries.
お気に入りの音楽を聴くことで，気持ちが落ち着き，心配事を忘れることができます。

Exercising, like jogging or cycling, is my way of releasing stress.
ジョギングやサイクリングなどの運動が，私のストレス解消法です。

Chapter 9 Stress **75**

Chapter 10

Mindfulness

「今，この瞬間」に集中することで様々な良い効果がもたらされるといわれているマインドフルネスについて学びます。

Introduction

どんな時に頭が空っぽになり，「今，この瞬間」に集中することができますか？ いろいろな方法を探してみましょう。

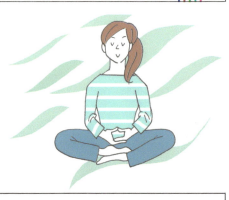

マインドフルネスの実践方法
ユニークなものや文化の違いによるものも探してみましょう。

自身が実践して効果があったものをシェアしましょう。

10-1. Dialogue

Riku（R）と Megu（M）が学食で話しています。

R: Do you ever feel irritable or get stressed and depressed?

M: Yes, quite often actually. Daily university classes and assignments are stressful, and thinking about the upcoming national exams sometimes makes me depressed.

R: I've been feeling a lot of stress lately too. I often end up escaping reality by using my smartphone for long periods of time. Because of that, my eyes and brain get tired, and when I finally try to study, I can't concentrate.

M: I understand how you feel. I recently heard that mindfulness can help with stress relief and even have positive effects on mood and depression.

R: I've heard of mindfulness before, but what does it mean?

M: Mindfulness is a noun made by adding "ness" to the adjective "mindful," which means attentive or aware. Here, we will keep it as simple as possible: "to focus one's awareness on the here and now," or you can think of it as "emptying your mind." It originally started as a part of religion, but now, through development and evolution, it is seen as a kind of stress reduction exercise popular in the West.

R: I'm not good at exercising regularly, though.

M: That's okay. There are practices that only take about five minutes a day.

R: In that case, maybe I can do it!

M: Personally, I spend about five minutes every day during my commute, before bed, or in the bath, just focusing on my breathing. It really helps clear my mind.

---

feel irritable
イライラを感じる

get stressed
ストレスを感じる

get depressed
気分が落ち込む

end up escaping
結局, 現実逃避してしまう

mindfulness
マインドフルネス

focus one's awareness on～
～に意識を集中させる

the here and now
今この瞬間

clear one's mind
心を落ち着かせる

Chapter 10 Mindfulness **77**

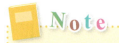

> マインドフルネスとは「今，この瞬間」に意識を集中させ，ありのままを受け入れる心の状態のことです。呼吸や感覚に集中することでストレスを減らし，心を落ち着ける効果があるといわれています。

Point　get + 過去分詞

get + 過去分詞（stressed）は「ストレスを感じる」「ストレスの状態になる」といった意味で，過去分詞が状態を表す形容詞として使われています。また，get + 過去分詞（depressed）は「気分が落ち込む」「憂鬱な気分である」という意味で，こちらも過去分詞が形容詞として使われている例です。

例1：I always get stressed before a big presentation.
　　　大きなプレゼンテーションの前は，いつもストレスを感じる。

例2：She got depressed after hearing the bad news.
　　　彼女は悪い知らせを聞いて，気分が落ち込んだ。

Drill

次の英文の［　］内の語句を並び替えて，日本語訳に合う英文にしなさい。

1. Lack of ［ feel / irritable / makes / me / sleep ］ and unable to concentrate.
   睡眠不足でイライラして集中できなくなる。

2. Not ［ regularly / get / makes / depressed / me / exercising ］ and feel low on energy.
   定期的に運動しないと気分が落ち込みエネルギーが低く感じる。

3. Eating junk food ［ up / you / making / end / gain / can ］ weight.
   ジャンクフードを食べると，最終的に体重が増える可能性がある。

4. I ［ activities / on / my / energy / focus ］ that make me feel relaxed like meditation.
   リラックスできる活動，たとえば瞑想にエネルギーを集中させている。

5. Mindfulness practice ［ me / and / helps / stay / the here / in ］ now and reduce stress.
   マインドフルネスを実践することで今この瞬間に集中しストレスを減らす。

Questions and Answers Q&A

会話文を読み，次の問に英語で答えなさい。

1. What happens to Riku when he uses his smartphone for long periods of time?

2. What can produce positive effects on mood and depression?

3. What does Megu do in the bath to relieve stress?

10-2. Reading

Vocabulary

alleviate	軽減する	conscious	意識している
anxiety	不安	depression	うつ病
bodily sensation	身体感覚	insomnia	不眠
breathing	呼吸	meditation	瞑想
chronic back pain	慢性的な腰痛	standard care	標準ケア
clinical medicine	臨床医学	treatment	治療
cognitive-behavioral therapy (CBT)	認知行動療法		

Have you ever heard of the term "mindfulness"? Mindfulness is derived from the adjective mindful, which means "aware or attentive." By adding "ness", it becomes a noun that translates to "(the state of) being conscious." In simple terms, it can be defined as focusing awareness on the present moment. Alternatively, it could be described as emptying your mind. In mindfulness, the focus is on breathing and bodily sensations, making an effort to concentrate on the "now" rather than the past or future.

When people hear mindfulness, many might think of practices like meditation, yoga, or Zen Buddhism. For example, in Zen, seated

be derived from
～から派生した

Chapter 10 Mindfulness **79**

meditation (*zazen*) is common, focusing on posture, breathing, and concentrating on the present moment. However, in recent years, the religious aspects have been set aside, and people are practicing mindfulness in various ways in their daily lives. Mindfulness is being implemented in fields such as education, healthcare, business, and sports, gaining popularity in many countries. It's also well-known that world-class athletes incorporate elements of mindfulness into their mental training.

So, what exactly is this "mindfulness," said to help reduce daily stress and improve sports performance? First, let's take a look at a case where mindfulness was introduced as a stress reduction method on a university's homepage. On Southern Utah University's website, four breathing techniques are introduced, including one that involves closing one nostril. The website claims that by focusing your attention on your breath, you can clear your mind of distractions and bring your mind to a state of emptiness. Another example of this is called sensory exercises, where you concentrate on the physical sensation of water on your hands or soft texture of a stuffed animal and focus your awareness on those sensations.

In Brazil, there was a study where university students participated in eight 90-minute mindfulness sessions. While no significant effect was observed in the anxiety category, improvements were noted in stress, depression, and insomnia. In another study, Cherkin et al. (2016) compared three types of treatments: mindfulness, cognitive-behavioral therapy (CBT), and standard care, to see which was more effective in reducing chronic back pain. The results showed that mindfulness, like cognitive-behavioral therapy, significantly reduced chronic back pain when compared to standard care. Both treatments were more effective than standard care in reducing pain, with the benefits lasting for 26 weeks.

As we've seen, mindfulness is being actively studied in both educational settings and clinical medicine. Why not try alleviating your worries and stress with simple mindfulness practices, like focusing on your breathing or the sensations in your hands?

Point 💡 受動態の進行形

「be ＋ being ＋過去分詞」の形をとり，「今まさに実行されている・導入されつつある」ことを表します。

A new policy is being discussed by the government.
新しい政策が政府によって議論されつつある。

Drill ✏️

次の英文の［　　］内の語句を並び替えて，日本語訳に合う英文にしなさい。

1. Modern jazz ［ variety / of / a / derived / is / from ］ African American musical traditions.
   現代ジャズは様々なアフリカ系アメリカ人の音楽的伝統から派生している。

   _____

2. New health policies ［ implemented / are / to / healthier / being / promote ］ lifestyle.
   健康的なライフスタイルを促進するために，新しい健康政策が実施されている。

   _____

3. She ［ work / about / aside / worries / set / her ］ to focus on her health.
   彼女は健康に集中するために，仕事の悩みをいったん忘れることにした。

   _____

4. Eating foods rich in vitamins and minerals, ［ vegetables / and / such / fruits / as ］, can boost your immune system.
   果物や野菜など，ビタミンやミネラルが豊富な食べ物を食べることで，免疫システムを強化することができる。

   _____

5. The new diet plan ［ on / had / a / significant / effect ］ overall health.
   新しいダイエットプランは，健康全般に顕著な効果をもたらした。

   _____

Chapter 10 Mindfulness **81**

Summary

1〜5に入る適切な語句を選択肢から選び，本文の要約を完成させなさい。

マインドフルネスは，1) _____ や身体感覚に注意を向けることで「今この瞬間」を意識することに焦点を当てた実践である。呼吸法や感覚に集中するエクササイズを通じて，心を落ち着かせ，ストレスを2) _____ するのに役立つ。研究によれば，マインドフルネスはストレス，うつ，3) _____ の症状を改善し，4) _____ と同様に慢性的な5) _____ を軽減する効果があることが示されている。

選択肢： 痛み 軽減 不眠 呼吸 認知行動療法

Questions and Answers

本文を読み，次の問に英語で答えなさい。

1. In mindfulness, what should you concentrate on rather than the past or future?

_____

2. In what fields has mindfulness been implemented outside of religious practices?

_____

3. What is well-known about world-class athletes?

_____

4. What example of a mindfulness technique is used at Southern Utah University?

_____

5. What were the findings of the mindfulness study conducted in Brazil?

_____

Activity

マインドフルネスや瞑想，呼吸法を使って，雑念を取り払い「今，この瞬間」に集中してみましょう。どの方法が一番集中しやすいか，みんなで話し合いましょう。また，うまくいかない時にどんな理由で失敗するのかも一緒に考えてみましょう。

参考例：

1. **深呼吸**：ゆっくりと深く呼吸し，息を吸う時と吐く時に意識を集中します。鼻から吸って，口から吐く方法が効果的です。

2. **ボディスキャン**：体の各部位に意識を向け，リラックスさせていきます。足から頭まで，順番に意識を集中していきます。

3. **視覚的焦点**：一つの物に集中して，その形や色，質感に意識を向けます。例えば，キャンドルの炎や自然の景色などを見てみましょう。

4. **数を数える**：息を吸いながら1，吐きながら2，というように呼吸に合わせて数を数えます。頭を空っぽにして集中しやすくなります。

5. **マインドフルウォーキング**：ゆっくり歩きながら，足が地面につく感覚や体の動きに集中します。歩くことに全神経を使うことで，心が落ち着きます。

6. **音に集中する**：周りの音を聴いて，その音に意識を集中させます。音楽や自然の音（風，鳥の声など）を聴くのも良い方法です。

7. **瞑想アプリの使用**：瞑想のガイドを提供するアプリを検索し，リラックスした状態を作り出します。

8. **5-4-3-2-1法**：目の前にあるものを，5つ見つけ，4つ触れ，3つ聴き，2つ匂い，1つ味わいます。

Chapter 10 Mindfulness　**83**

Chapter 11

Broaden Your Horizons

世界に目を向け，自分の視野を広げるためのヒントについて学びます。

Introduction

今後訪れてみたい国はありますか。その国におけるマナーや常識などについて調べてまとめましょう。

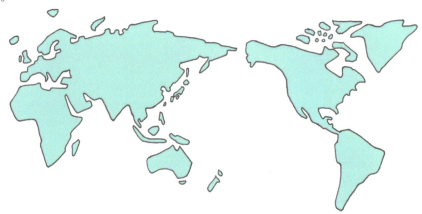

訪れてみたい国

その国におけるマナーや常識

11-1. Dialogue

放課後, Megu (M) と Haruto (H) はカフェで将来について話しています。

H: What are your plans after you graduate from university?

> graduate from〜
> 〜を卒業する

M: I'm going to work as a nurse at a local hospital.

H: Have you thought about working abroad?

M: Once I gain experience working in a Japanese hospital and save some money, I want to go to graduate school in the U.S. to become a Nurse Practitioner (NP) and provide more advanced and specialized care. How about you?

H: After I get used to working in a hospital in Japan, I actually plan to do medical volunteer work as a nurse abroad.

M: I see. What kind of organizations are involved in that?

> be involved in〜
> 〜に関わる

H: A well-known one is Médecins Sans Frontières (MSF), a private organization founded in France in 1971. It provides medical aid to areas affected by conflicts and natural disasters in an independent, neutral, and impartial manner. Another is the Youth Overseas Cooperation Volunteers, dispatched by the Japan International Cooperation Agency (JICA). It has been active since 1965, not only in the medical field, but in the educational, agricultural, forestry, and fishery fields as well, all across the world.

> found 設立する
>
> provide 提供する
>
> conflict 紛争
>
> natural disaster
> 自然災害
>
> impartial 公平な
>
> dispatch 派遣する

M: You'll be able to use your expertise to help people in other countries.

> expertise 専門的知識

H: But there are also things you can do right here in Japan. The number of foreign residents in Japan is increasing every year, so it is necessary to provide support tailored to each culture and religion.

> resident 居住者
>
> (be) tailored to〜
> 〜に合わせた

M: I'd like to try volunteering while I'm a student to help children

Chapter 11 Broaden Your Horizons **85**

from other cultural backgrounds with their homework. In addition, I want to focus on improving my English for smoother communication.

smooth　円滑な

H: I will do my best, too! It will not only broaden my horizons but also expand my field of activity.

broaden one's horizons
〜の視野を広げる

 動詞の「ing」

現在分詞と動名詞の2種類があります。

1. 現在分詞

be動詞とともに用い，動作が進行していることを表します。
The number of foreign residents in Japan is increasing every year.
日本の在留外国人数は毎年増加している。

限定用法では，名詞の前後につき，形容詞的な役割を果たします。
Once I gain experience working in a Japanese hospital, I plan to work abroad.
日本の病院で働く経験を積んだら海外で働くつもりです。

※ただし「〜するための」という意味で名詞の前につく場合は，動名詞です。
例：洗うための機械（洗濯機）＝ washing machine, 炒めるための平なべ（フライパン）＝ frying pan

2. 動名詞

名詞的な役割を果たします。前置詞の後は，名詞・動名詞しか置くことができません。この場合はaboutという前置詞に続けるために動名詞が用いられています。
Have you thought about working abroad?
海外で働くことについて考えたことはあるか。

Drill

空欄に入る適切な語句を選択肢から選び記号で書きなさい。

1. Volunteering helps us (　　　).

2. Policies should (　　　) meet the needs of the people.

3. Various organizations (　　　) providing medical aid to people.

4. All the medical professionals (　　　) medical universities.

5. Climate change has led to an increase in (　　　).

(a) resident	(b) broaden our horizons
(d) are involved in	(e) natural disasters

(c) graduated from
(f) be tailored to

Questions and Answers

会話文を読み，次の問に英語で答えなさい。

1. Complete the chart.

	MSF	JICA
設立年		
設立国		
活動内容		
活動地域		

2. What kind of support should be provided for foreign residents living in Japan?

Chapter 11 Broaden Your Horizons　87

11-2. Reading

Vocabulary

accurate	正確な	insult	侮辱
acquaintance	知り合い	lingua franca	共通語
antioxidant	抗酸化物質	mindful	心を配って
appropriate	適切な	offend	感情を害する
consider	みなす	permissible	許される
consume	消費する	recognize	認識する
conversely	反対に	region	地域
define	定義する	religious	宗教の
definition	定義	restriction	制限
dietary	食事の	sacred	神聖な
encounter	に出会う	treat	遇する
forbid	を禁ずる	unintentionally	意図せず
guarantee	保証する		

English is recognized as a global lingua franca, spoken by approximately 1.5 billion people when counting both native and second-language speakers. Now, does this mean knowing English alone guarantees accurate communication with people worldwide? The answer is no. This is because each of us has a uniquely different cultural background. There are various definitions of culture, but Ishii et al. (2013) define it as "the common ways of thinking, behaving, seeing, and dealing with things that are considered 'normal' within the group or region where one belongs". In other words, even if we speak a common language like English, miscommunication can arise due to cultural differences. While it is impossible to learn about every culture around the world, we need to at least recognize this fact.

What does "cultural difference" mean? The easiest example is food culture. In both Japan and the Philippines, people eat rice

be recognized as〜
〜として認識されている

, spoken　分詞構文

deal with〜
〜に対応する

due to〜　〜が原因で

porridge when they are sick, but the people in the Philippines add chicken and heaps of ginger to it. In Finland, some people consume soup made from bilberries, a type of berry rich in antioxidants. Religious dietary restrictions also vary. In Hinduism, cows are widely believed to be sacred, so Hindus are forbidden from eating beef. In Islam, pork and alcohol are forbidden, so Muslims consume halal food, which is food regarded as permissible according to God.

　Gestures also differ across cultures. Take the peace sign, for example, familiar in Japan when taking photos. In the United Kingdoms and Australia, showing the back of your hand while making the peace sign is an insult, so be careful. Similarly, in Singapore and Thailand, pointing the soles of your shoes at someone is thought to be highly insulting. It's essential to be mindful not to unintentionally offend others.

Communication styles also differ. For instance, the appropriate way to treat someone you've just met varies between "peach cultures" and "coconut cultures". In "peach cultures" like the United States and Brazil, it is appropriate to smile at new acquaintances, share personal information, and ask personal questions. Conversely, in "coconut cultures" like Germany and France, such behavior is reserved for close relationships. Thus, misunderstandings are likely to occur between them, even if they speak fluent English.

　If you, as a future healthcare professional, encounter people connected to foreign countries domestically or internationally, please remember not to judge their words and actions based on your own cultural norms. Instead, as you engage with them, consider that their cultural norms may differ from yours.

---

heaps of〜　沢山の〜

（be）made from〜
〜から作られた

（be）rich in〜
〜が豊富である

be regarded as〜
〜とみなされる

according to〜
〜に従って

engage with〜
〜と関わる

differ from〜
〜と異なる

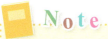

桃文化とココナッツ文化

「桃文化」では初対面の人に対する対応は桃の果肉ように柔らかいが，本当の自分は硬い種の中に隠されているといわれています。「ココナッツ文化」では初対面の人に対する対応はココナッツの殻のように硬いが，いったん仲良くなると打ち解けるといわれています。

Point 💡 分詞構文

分詞構文は「接続詞＋主語＋動詞」の代わりに，「コンマ＋ 現在分詞／過去分詞」を用いて文を簡潔にします。例文の場合，主節に状況説明を加えています。また，「〜される」と受け身の意味になる場合に過去分詞を使います。

例：English is recognized as a global lingua franca, <u>spoken</u> by approximately 1.5 billion people.
英語は世界の共通語として認識され，およそ15億人によって話されている。

Drill ✏️

[　　] 内の語句を並び替えて，日本語訳に合う英文にしなさい。

1. [in / is / diversity / rich / the world] .
世界は多様性に富んでいる。

_____

2. It is important [appropriately / to / with / each / deal / situation] .
それぞれの状況に適切に対処することは重要だ。

_____

3. Cultural values [group / to / from / differ / another / often / one] .
文化的な価値観はグループによってしばしば異なる。

_____

4. English [tool / for / regarded / information / important / as / is / accessing / an] globally.
英語は世界の情報にアクセスするための重要な手段とみなされている。

_____

5. [essential / diverse / is / engaging / opening / for / with / viewpoints] our minds.
多様な視点に触れることは，心を開くために不可欠だ。

_____

Summary 📝

1～6に入る適切な語句を選択肢から選び，本文の要約を完成させなさい。

　英語は世界の1) ＿＿＿＿＿＿＿＿とされているが，英語力だけでは他国の人々と正確な2) ＿＿＿＿＿＿＿が図れるとはいえない。なぜならそれぞれの3) ＿＿＿＿＿＿＿が異なるためである。文化とは特定のグループや地域などで当たり前とされている共通の考え方や行動の仕方である。具体例としては食文化，ジェスチャー，4) ＿＿＿＿＿＿＿の違いが挙げられる。4) ＿＿＿＿＿＿＿では，初対面の人に対する適切な接し方の違いがある。「桃文化」では笑顔や5) ＿＿＿＿＿＿＿の開示が一般的だが，「ココナッツ文化」ではこのような接し方は親しい友人に限定される。したがって，自分の6) ＿＿＿＿＿＿＿をもとに他の人々の言動を判断・評価しないことが重要である。

選択肢：	文化的背景	個人情報	意思疎通	常識
	コミュニケーションスタイル		共通語	

Questions and Answers 🅠🅐

本文を読み，次の問に英語で答えなさい。

1. How is culture defined?

   _____

2. What do people from the Philippines and Finland eat when they get sick?

   _____

3. What are the two examples of offensive gestures?

   _____

4. What is the suitable communication style for individuals from a peach culture when they encounter new people?

   _____

5. What should you avoid doing when you become a healthcare professional?

   _____

Chapter 11 Broaden Your Horizons **91**

Activity

あなたの地元またはあなたが通う大学の地域に暮らす外国の方について，国籍や人数，住民全体に占める割合などを調べましょう。また，そのうちの1ヶ国を選び，その国の言語や文化，生活様式などについてまとめましょう。さらに，それらをもとに，医療職に就いた時にケアを提供するうえで配慮すべき点について考えましょう。

地域に暮らす外国の方

使用言語や文化，生活様式など（1ヶ国を選択）

ケアを提供するうえで配慮すべき点

Chapter 12

Volunteer Activity

ボランティアの歴史，意味，活動内容について学びます。

Introduction

ボランティア活動にはどのような種類がありますか？

例）高校でどのようなボランティア活動の経験をしたのかについて，グループで話しましょう。

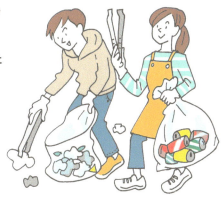

12-1. Dialogue

Haruto（H）と Megu（M）は特別養護老人ホームでのボランティアについて話しています。

H: Hello. I've gathered you all here today to ask for your help with the volunteer work I'm currently involved in.

ask for　求める

M: We don't know what kind of volunteer work you want us to help out with, so could you explain that to us first?

you want us to
私達に〜してもらいたい

H: Sure thing. I'm currently volunteering to read books at a nursing home. Since there are some people at the nursing home who have difficulty reading books by themselves, I read their favorite books to them.

nursing home
特別養護老人ホーム

by themselves
彼ら自身で（自分で）

M: Is it difficult for them to read due to illness?

due to　〜のために

H: I'm not entirely sure, but they really appreciate it when I sit next to them and read the books they request.

appreciate　感謝する

M: That's a great activity, but these days there are audio books available on tapes and CDs, as well as online resources. Wouldn't it be good for them to listen to those?

available　利用可能

...as well as〜
〜ばかりではなく…も

H: That's true. Professional narrators are involved in those, so they are very good at reading. However, it seems that sitting next to a person and having various conversations while reading a book are more enjoyable for them.

are very good at 〜ing
〜することがとてもうまい

M: Engaging in live conversations is indeed enjoyable. Communication between people is absolutely necessary.

H: Exactly. It's important not to just engage in activities mechanically but to enjoy human interaction as well.

not A but B
AではなくBをする

M: So it's not just about reading books, but also about having conversations.

H: That's right. Just listening to their stories makes them very happy. So we listen to their stories, have conversations, and if they wish, read books to them too. I would love to follow your advice and join in on this volunteer activity.

make ~ very happy
~をとても幸せにする
makeは使役動詞

M: Me too!

H: I'm happy to hear that. Let's think together about what we can do to work together on this activity.

what we can do
私達ができること
whatは先行詞を含む関係
代名詞。～のこと, ～のもの

Point 💡

A as well as B：Bだけではなく A も～
➡ Bから逆に訳す。動詞は A にかかってくる。
　You as well as I are a college student.
　私だけではなくあなたも大学生です。

are very good at ~ing：～することがとてもうまい
　She is good at singing.
　彼女は歌うのが上手です。
　He is good at playing the piano.
　彼はピアノを演奏するのが上手です。

not A but B：A ではなく B が～
　In this area, not young people but elderly people do a lot of volunteer activities.
　この地域では，若者ではなく高齢者が多くのボランティア活動をします。

Drill ✏️

以下の文章を英語に訳しなさい。

1. 私の母は料理が得意です。

_____

2. トムだけではなくメアリーも看護学科の学生です。（as well as を用いて）

_____

3. 彼らは洋食ではなく和食が好きです。

_____

Chapter 12　Volunteer Activity　**95**

Questions and Answers

会話文を読み，次の問に英語で答えなさい。

1. What has Haruto been doing at the nursing home recently?
   _____
2. When do the elderly people enjoy?
   _____
3. What is it that Haruto thinks is important to do?
   _____

12-2. Reading

Vocabulary

academic years	学年度	initially	最初に，冒頭に
autonomy	自主性	international cooperation	国際協力
boundary	境界線，限界		
child-rearing	子どもの養育	nature conservation	自然保護
company employees	会社の従業員	participation	参加
department	学科	proactively	先取りして，事前対策として
disaster victims	被災者	self-defense group	自己防衛集団
emerge	明らかになる，出てくる	span	（期間，範囲に）わたる
engage in	～に従事する，没頭する	spontaneity	自主性
enhance	高める，増す	voluntarily	自発的に，自分の意思で
fundraising	募金	voluntus or volo	ボランティアの語源
genders	性，ジェンダー		

Everyone is familiar with the term "volunteer" and some people may have even participated in volunteer activities themselves. Such activities include helping at local festivals, assisting with fundraising activities, helping elder people and cleaning up the beach. Let's start by understanding what volunteer means. The term volunteer was first used in England in the 17th century, referring to a "self-defense group protecting their community" or "people who raised their hands to participate in activities." The origin of the word volunteer comes from the Latin word voluntus or volo, meaning "free will," "doing something voluntarily," and "willingly doing something," focusing on the aspect of acting voluntarily for people or society. Additionally, the concept of unpaid work emerged, where individuals engage in activities at their own expense to further meet societal needs and be helpful.

When the word "volunteer" was introduced to Japan, it was translated as service activity and used differently from its original meaning. Concepts like autonomy and spontaneity were replaced with the notion of good deeds. Therefore, volunteering in Japan was initially thought to be limited to welfare activities. Today, however, it spans various fields, including not only welfare, but healthcare, education, international exchange, international cooperation, sports, and the arts. Until the 1970s, young people were the ones primarily involved in volunteering in Japan. From the 1980s, however, the participation of middle-aged and older women increased, and following the 1995 Great Hanshin-Awaji Earthquake, students, company employees, retirees, and people of a wide range of ages and genders began participating in volunteer activities.

Types of volunteer activities include:

1. Child-rearing support
2. Nature conservation and environmental protection
3. Support for disaster victims
4. Assistance to the elderly and disabled
5. Organizing and managing events and social activities
6. International exchange

All of these are important activities.

The additional benefits of volunteering through a university in specific include:

1. Interacting with others beyond the boundaries of academic years and departments
2. Having experiences with the regional community, environmental issues, and taking care of local children
3. Having various interactions and gaining different experiences through volunteer opportunities outside the university

interacting with others
他の人との交流

gaining 得ること

opportunity 機会

During their school years, students can enhance their planning, communication, and problem-solving skills not only through academics, but also by proactivity taking part in volunteer activities that address various social issues. Let's convey the spirit of volunteering to create a better society, with individual efforts. The essential aspects of volunteering are:

convey 知らせる, 伝える

1. Protecting secrets
2. Keeping promises
3. Understanding what is right and wrong as a human being
4. Not accepting money or goods
5. Taking responsibility for one's actions and words

Questions and Answers Q A

本文を読み，次の問に英語で答えなさい。

1. Where does the origin of the word "volunteer" come from?

_____

2. What was volunteering initially thought to refer to?

_____

3. What type of volunteer activities are mentioned in the reading?

_____

4. What are the additional benefits of volunteering through a university?

_____

5. What are the essential aspects of volunteering?

_____

Summary 📄

1〜10に入る適切な語句を選択肢から選び，本文の要約を完成させなさい。

　「ボランティア」という言葉は1)＿＿＿＿＿＿＿＿に2)＿＿＿＿＿＿＿で使われ始め，「自分たちの地域を自分たちで守る3)＿＿＿＿＿＿＿」または「自分で活動に手を挙げた4)＿＿＿＿＿＿＿」の意味があった。volunteerの語源はラテン語の voluntus であり，さらに"volo"ともいわれていた。日本にvolunteerという言葉が入ってきたとき，日本語の訳が「5)＿＿＿＿＿＿＿」となったため本来の意味とは異なって使用されるようになった。「6)＿＿＿＿＿＿＿」「自発性」から「善い行い」の考えが広がった。日本では1970年代までは7)＿＿＿＿＿＿＿が中心的に活動していたが，8)＿＿＿＿＿＿＿に入ると中高年の9)＿＿＿＿＿＿＿の参加が増え，1995年の阪神・淡路大震災を契機にして学生，10)＿＿＿＿＿＿＿，退職者など男女幅広い年齢の人がボランティア活動に参加するようになった。

選択肢：	アメリカ	義勇兵	若者	高齢者	1980年代	20世紀
	会社員	自主性	イギリス	17世紀	自警団	フランス
	20世紀	奉仕活動	女性			

Activity 👍

大学で行いたいボランティア活動について話し合いましょう。大学ボランティアセンターにはいろいろなボランティア活動の情報がありますので，参考にしてください。

Chapter 12 Volunteer Activity　**99**

参考文献

Chapter1

Dialogue

Aaker, J. & Bagdonas, N. (2020). Humour, Seriously: Why Humour is a Superpower at work and in life. Portfolio Penguin.

Hayashi, K., Hayashi, T., Iwanaga, S., et al. (2003). Laughter lowered the increase in postprandial blood glucose. *Diabetes Care*, 26(5), 1651-1652.

安藤貞雄 (2005). 現代英文法講義. 開拓社.

伊丹仁朗, 昇幹夫, 手嶋秀毅 (1994). 笑いと免疫能. 心身医学, 34(7), 565-571.

大平哲也 (2023). 1日1回！大笑いの健康医学. さくら舎.

大平哲也 (2012). 笑うと血圧が下がる？「笑い」と「高血圧・循環器系疾患」との関連について. 公衆衛生, 76, 649-652.

大平哲也 (2015). 笑い等のポジティブな心理介入が生活習慣病発症・重症化予防に及ぼす影響についての疫学研究, 平成26年度 総括・分担研究報告書, 国立研究開発法人国立がん研究センター. がん情報サービス：最新がん統計のまとめ https://ganjoho.jp/reg_stat/statistics/stat/summary.html

Reading

Gill, J., Endres-Brocks, J., Bauer, P., et al. (1987). The effect of ABO blood group on the diagnosis of von Willebrand Disease. *Blood*., 69(6), 1691-1695.

Takayama, W., Endo, A., Koguchi, H., et al. (2018). The impact of blood type O on mortality of severe trauma patients: a retrospective observational study. *Crit Care*, 22(1), 100.

安藤貞雄 (2005). 現代英文法講義. 開拓社.

医療情報科学研究所編 (2017). 病気が見える vol.5 血液 第2版. メディックメディア.

髙木久代編著 (2018). やさしいメディカル英語. 講談社.

Chapter2

髙木久代編著 (2018). やさしいメディカル英語. 講談社.

坂井建雄, 河原克雅 (2021). カラー図解 人体の正常構造と機能【全10巻縮刷版】改訂第4版. 日本医事新報社.

Barbara Janson Cohen (2011). Medical Terminology: An illustrated Guide Sixth Edition. Wolters Kluwer | Lippincott Williams & Wilkins.

佐藤達夫, 松尾理 (2009). みえる人体：構造・機能・病態. 南江堂.

Chapter3

Dialogue

United Nations. (2023). International Day of Clean Air for Blue Skies, 7 September. https://www.un.org/en/observances/clean-air-day

World Health Organization. (2023). Air Pollution: The Invisible Health Threat. https://www.who.int/news-room/feature-stories/detail/air-pollution--the-invisible-health-threat

World Health Organization. (2022). Ambient (outdoor) Air Pollution. https://www.who.int/news-room/fact-sheets/detail/ambient-(outdoor)-air-quality-and-healt

World Health Organization. Air Quality, Energy and Health: Types of Pollutants. https://www.who.int/teams/environment-climate-change-and-health/air-quality-and-health/health- impacts/types-of-pollutants

安藤貞雄（2005）．現代英文法講義．開拓社．

Reading

Cleveland Clinic. Mouth Breathing: What It Is, Complications & Treatments. https://my.clevelandclinic.org/health/diseases/22734-mouth-breathing

Nogami, Y., Saitoh, I., Inada, E., et al. (2021). Prevalence of an incompetent lip seal during growth periods throughout Japan: a large-scale, survey-based, cross-sectional study. *Environmental Health and Preventive Medicine*, 26(11). https://environhealthprevmed.biomedcentral.com/articles/10.1186/s12199-021-00933-5

安藤貞雄（2005）．現代英文法講義．開拓社．

一般社団法人日本呼吸器学会．呼吸器Q＆A：Q13　呼吸が速くなります。過換気だと言われました．https://www.jrs.or.jp/citizen/faq/q13.html

今井一彰・中島潤子（2021）．世界一簡単な驚きの健康法マウステーピング．幻冬舎．

医療情報科学研究所編（2013）．病気が見えるvol.4 呼吸器　第2版．メディックメディア．

さいたま赤十字病院看護部編（2021）．本当に大切なことが1冊でわかる呼吸器．照林社．

髙木久代編著（2018）．やさしいメディカル英語．講談社．

西原克成（2010）．アレルギー体質は口呼吸が原因だった．青春出版社．

日本医師会．深呼吸をしましょう：腹式呼吸のやり方．https://www.med.or.jp/komichi/holiday/sports_02.html

Chapter4

髙木久代編著（2018）．やさしいメディカル英語．講談社．

坂井建雄・橋本尚詞（2012）．ぜんぶわかる人体解剖図．成美堂出版．

MSDマニュアル家庭版：過敏性腸症候群（IBS）03.消化器系の病気 - MSDマニュアル家庭版

Chapter 5

髙木久代編著（2018）．やさしいメディカル英語．講談社．

坂井建雄・橋本尚詞（2012）．ぜんぶわかる人体解剖図．成美堂出版．

豊永 彰（2009）．英文法ビフォー＆アフター．南雲堂．

Chapter 6

髙木久代編著（2018）．やさしいメディカル英語．講談社．

Chapter 7

豊永 彰（2009）．英文法ビフォー＆アフター．南雲堂．

公益財団法人長寿科学振興財団．健康長寿ネット．薬と食べ物の相互作用 https://www.tyojyu.or.jp/net/kenkou-tyoju/eiyou-shippei/yobou-kusuri-shokuji.html

Chapter 8

髙木久代（2023）．はじめての薬膳．かざひの出版．

日本薬膳学会（2024）．和の薬膳．講談社．

Chapter 9

厚生労働省 平成22年国民生活基礎調査の概況 悩みやストレスの状況．https://www.mhlw.go.jp/toukei/saikin/hw/k-tyosa/k-tyosa10/3-3.html

増谷文雄（1985）．この人を見よ ブッダ・ゴータマの生涯．講談社．

Chapter 10

大谷彰（2014）．マインドフルネス入門講義．金剛出版．

Gallo, G. G., et al. (2023). A randomized controlled trial of mindfulness: effects on university students' mental health. *International Journal of Mental Health Systems*. 17(32).

Cherkin, Daniel C., et al. (2016). Effect of Mindfulness-Based Stress Reduction vs Cognitive Behavioral Therapy or Usual Care on Back Pain and Functional Limitations in Adults with Chronic Low Back Pain: A Randomized Clinical Trial. *JAMA*. 315(12). 1240-1249.

Savannah Byers (2021). Seven Mindfulness Techniques for College Students. Southern Utah University. https://www.suu.edu/blog/2021/10/mindfulness-techniques-students.html

Chapter 11

Dialogue

安藤貞雄（2005）．現代英文法講義．開拓社．

国境なき医師団　https://www.msf.or.jp/about/

JICA 青年海外協力隊　https://www.jica.go.jp/volunteer/

Reading

Ethnologue. (2024). What are the top 200 most spoken languages?
　https://www.ethnologue.com/insights/ethnologue200/

Mayer, E. (2014). The Cultural Map: Breaking Through the Invisible Boundaries of Global
　Business. Public Affairs.

Ro, H. (2016). Here's what people from around the world eat when they are sick. Business
　Insider. June 23．https://www.businessinsider.com/what-people-from-around-the-world-
　eat-when-they-are-sick-2016-6

Trompenaars, F& Hampden-Turner, C.(2008). Riding the Waves of Culture: Understanding
　Diversity in Global Business. Nicholas Brealey Publishing.

安藤貞雄（2005）．現代英文法講義．開拓社．

石井敏・久米昭元・長谷川典子・桜木敏行・石黒武人（2013）．はじめて学ぶ異文化コミュ
　ニケーション．有斐閣選書．

一般社団法人ハラル・ジャパン協会．ハラル（ハラール）基礎知識．https://jhba.jp/halal/

デスモンド・モリス著・東山安子訳（1999）．ボディトーク 新装版：世界の身ぶり辞典．
　三省堂．

八代京子・荒木晶子・樋口容視子・山本志都・コミサロフ喜美（2001）．異文化コミュニケ
　ーションワークブック．三修社．

Chapter 12

二宮雅也（2017）．スポーツボランティア読本．悠光堂

厚生労働省社会・援護局．ボランティアについて．https://www.mhlw.go.jp/shingi/2007/
　12/dl/s1203-5e_0001.pdf

東京ボランティア・市民活動センター．ボランティア活動, 4つの原則．https://www.tvac.
　or.jp/shiru/hajime/gensoku.html

索引

英文

AED	10
airway	21
antibiotics	55
anus	29
anxiety	72
aorta	12
appetite	69
arterial blood	12
atrioventricular node	12
atrium	12
bladder	37
blood pressure	2
bone marrow	4, 46
breathing	79
bronchus	21
cancer cell	2
capillary	37
chest	21
chronic obstructive pulmonary disease	18
clinical medicine	79
cognitive-behavioral therapy	79
depression	79
depressive	72
detoxify	62
diabetes	2
diarrhea	27
dietary	88
electrocardiogram	12
endocrine gland	29
enzyme	55
esophagus	21
fatigue	69
frature	43
gastrointestinal	71

hemoglobin	4
heartbeat	12
high blood pressure	53
immune system	2
insomnia	79
insulin	29
intestine	29
kidney	37
ligament	46
liver	26
lobe	21
lymphocyte	2
medication	55
metabolize	55
must	3
nasal cavity	21
nutrition	60
oxygen	12
pancreas	29
pathogen	4
pollutant	18
pulmonary artery	12
religious	88
respiratory	18
side effect	55
sinoatrial node	12
sleep disorder	21
stomach	26
stroke	18
symptom	21
tendon	46
tissue	4
toxin	37
trachea	21
treatment	79
urethra	37
urine	37
vein	12
ventricle	12
vertebra	46

和文

あ行

胃腸の	71
うつ病	79
栄養	60
汚染物質	18

か行

がん細胞	2
気管	12
気道	21
胸部	21
血圧	2
血液	1
解毒する	62
下痢	27
腱	46
高血圧	53
抗生物質	55
酵素	55
肛門	29
呼吸	79
呼吸器系	17
骨格系	42
骨髄	4, 46
骨折	43

さ行

酸素	12
自動体外式除細動器	10
宗教の	88
消化器系	26
静脈	12
食事の	88
食道	21
食欲	69
心室	12
腎臓	37
靱帯	46
心電図	12
心拍	12

心房	12
膵臓	29
睡眠障害	21
組織	4
卒中	18

た行

代謝する	55
大動脈	12
治療	79
椎骨	46
洞房結節	12
糖尿病	2
動脈血	12
投薬	55
毒	37

な行

内分泌腺	29
尿	37
認知行動療法	79

は行

肺動脈	12
鼻腔	21
泌尿器系	34
病原体	4
疲労	69
不安	72
不眠	79
ヘモグロビン	4
膀胱	37
房室結節	12

ま・や・ら行

慢性閉塞性肺疾患	18
免疫系	2
毛細血管	37
抑うつの	72
臨床医学	79

編著者紹介

髙木久代
（たか ぎ ひさ よ）

鈴鹿医療科学大学 保健衛生学部 教授

NDC 490　　109p　　26cm

English for Anatomy and Mind
（イングリッシュ フォー ア ナ ト ミ ー アンド マインド）

2025年5月13日　第1刷発行

編著者	髙木久代（たか ぎ ひさ よ）
発行者	篠木和久
発行所	株式会社 講談社
	〒112-8001　東京都文京区音羽2-12-21
	販　売　(03)5395-5817
	業　務　(03)5395-3615

KODANSHA

編　集	株式会社 講談社サイエンティフィク
	代表　堀越俊一
	〒162-0825　東京都新宿区神楽坂2-14　ノービィビル
	編　集　(03)3235-3701
本文データ制作	鮎川　廉（アユカワデザインアトリエ）
本文印刷・製本	株式会社 ＫＰＳプロダクツ

落丁本・乱丁本は，購入書店名を明記のうえ，講談社業務宛にお送りください．
送料小社負担にてお取替えします．なお，この本の内容についてのお問い合わせは
講談社サイエンティフィク宛にお願いいたします．
定価はカバーに表示してあります．

© H. Takagi, 2025

本書のコピー，スキャン，デジタル化等の無断複製は著作権法上での例外を除き
禁じられています．本書を代行業者等の第三者に依頼してスキャンやデジタル化
することはたとえ個人や家庭内の利用でも著作権法違反です．

Printed in Japan

ISBN978-4-06-539717-6